WALe

Frederic P. Miller, Agnes F. Vandome,
John McBrewster (Ed.)

Retinitis Pigmentosa

Frederic P. Miller, Agnes F. Vandome,
John McBrewster (Ed.)

Retinitis Pigmentosa

Human eye, Nyctalopia, Tunnel vision,
Blindness, Dystrophy, Photoreceptor cell,
Retinal pigment epithelium, Retina,
Peripheral vision

Alphascript Publishing

Imprint

Publisher:
Alphascript Publishing is a trademark of
VDM Publishing House Ltd.,17 Rue Meldrum, Beau Bassin,1713-01 Mauritius
Email: info@vdm-publishing-house.com
Website: www.vdm-publishing-house.com

Published in 2011

Printed in: U.S.A., U.K., Germany. This book was not produced in Mauritius.

ISBN: 978-613-4-31648-4

Contents

Articles

References

Article Licenses

Retinitis pigmentosa

Retinitis pigmentosa	
Classification and external resources	
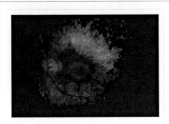 Fundus of patient with retinitis pigmentosa, mid stage (Bone spicule-shaped pigment deposits are present in the mid periphery along with retinal atrophy, while the macula is preserved although with a peripheral ring of depigmentation. Retinal vessels are attenuated.) From a review by Christian Hamel, 2006.	
ICD-10	H 35.5 [1]
ICD-9	362.74 [2]
OMIM	268000 [3]
MeSH	D012174 [4]

Retinitis pigmentosa (RP) is a group of genetic eye conditions that leads to incurable blindness.[5] In the progression of symptoms for RP, night blindness generally precedes tunnel vision by years or even decades. Many people with RP do not become legally blind until their 40s or 50s and retain some sight all their lives.[6] Others go completely blind from RP, in some cases as early as childhood. Progression of RP is different in each case.

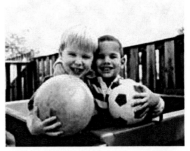

Normal vision. Courtesy NIH National Eye Institute

RP is a type of progressive retinal dystrophy, a group of inherited disorders in which abnormalities of the photoreceptors (rods and cones) or the retinal pigment epithelium (RPE) of the retina lead to progressive visual loss. Affected individuals first experience defective dark adaptation or nyctalopia (night blindness), followed by reduction of the peripheral visual field (known as tunnel vision) and, sometimes, loss of central vision late in the course of the disease.

Signs

Mottling of the retinal pigment epithelium with black *bone-spicule* pigmentation is typically indicative (or pathognomonic) of retinitis pigmentosa. Other ocular features include waxy pallor of the optic nerve head, attenuation (thinning) of the retinal vessels, cellophane maculopathy, cystic macular edema and posterior subcapsular cataract.

Diagnosis

The diagnosis of retinitis pigmentosa relies upon documentation of progressive loss in photoreceptor cell function by electroretinography (ERG) and visual field testing.

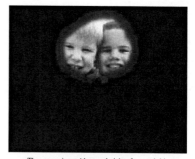

The same view with tunnel vision from retinitis pigmentosa. The blackness surrounding the central image does not indicate darkness, but rather a lack of perceived visual information.

The mode of inheritance of RP is determined by family history. At least 35 different genes or loci are known to cause "nonsyndromic RP" (RP that is not the result of another disease or part of a wider syndrome).

DNA testing is available on a clinical basis for:

- *RLBP1* [7] (autosomal recessive, Bothnia type RP)
- *RP1* [8] (autosomal dominant, RP1)
- *RHO* [9] (autosomal dominant, RP4)
- *RDS* [10] (autosomal dominant, RP7)
- *PRPF8* [11] (autosomal dominant, RP13)
- *PRPF3* [12] (autosomal dominant, RP18)
- CRB1 (autosomal recessive, RP12)
- *ABCA4* [13] (autosomal recessive, RP19)
- *RPE65* [14] (autosomal recessive, RP20)

For all other genes, molecular genetic testing is available on a research basis only.

RP can be inherited in an autosomal dominant, autosomal recessive, or X-linked manner. X-linked RP can be either recessive, affecting primarily only males, or dominant, affecting both males and females, although males are usually more mildly affected. Some digenic (controlled by two genes) and mitochondrial forms have also been described.

Genetic counseling depends on an accurate diagnosis, determination of the mode of inheritance in each family, and results of molecular genetic testing.

Associations

Retinitis pigmentosa is seen in a variety of diseases, so the differential of this sign alone, is broad.

- RP combined with deafness (congenital or progressive) is called Usher syndrome.
- RP combined with opthalmoplegia, dysphagia, ataxia, and cardiac conduction defects is seen in the mitochondrial DNA disorder Kearns-Sayre syndrome (aka Ragged Red Fiber Myopathy)
- RP combined with retardation, peripheral neuropathy, acanthotic (spiked) RBCs, ataxia, steatorrhea, is absence of VLDL is seen in abetalipoproteinemia.

Other conditions include neurosyphilis, toxoplasmosis(Emedicine "Retinitis Pigmentosa" [15]) and Refsum's disease.

Genetics

Retinitis pigmentosa (RP) is one of the most common forms of inherited retinal degeneration.[16] This disorder is characterized by the progressive loss of photoreceptor cells and may eventually lead to blindness.[17]

There are multiple genes that, when mutated, can cause the Retinitis pigmentosa phenotype.[18] In 1989, a mutation of the gene for rhodopsin, a pigment that plays an essential part in the visual transduction cascade enabling vision in low-light conditions, was identified. Since then, more than 100 mutations have been found in this gene, accounting for 15% of all types of retinal degeneration. Most of those mutations are missense mutations and inherited mostly in a dominant manner.

Types include:

OMIM	Gene	Type
180100 [19]	RP1	Retinitis pigmentosa-1
312600 [20]	RP2	Retinitis pigmentosa-2
300029 [21]	RPGR	Retinitis pigmentosa-3
608133 [22]	PRPH2	Retinitis pigmentosa-7
180104 [23]	RP9	Retinitis pigmentosa-9
180105 [24]	IMPDH1	Retinitis pigmentosa-10
600138 [25]	PRPF31	Retinitis pigmentosa-11
600105 [26]	CRB1	Retinitis pigmentosa-12, autosomal recessive
600059 [27]	PRPF8	Retinitis pigmentosa-13
600132 [28]	TULP1	Retinitis pigmentosa-14
600852 [29]	CA4	Retinitis pigmentosa-17
601414 [30]	HPRP3	Retinitis pigmentosa-18
601718 [31]	ABCA4	Retinitis pigmentosa-19
602772 [32]	EYS	Retinitis pigmentosa-25
608380 [33]	CERKL	Retinitis pigmentosa-26
607921 [34]	FSCN2	Retinitis pigmentosa-30
609923 [35]	TOPORS	Retinitis pigmentosa-31
610359 [36]	SNRNP200	Retinitis pigmentosa 33
610282 [37]	SEMA4A	Retinitis pigmentosa-35
610599 [38]	PRCD	Retinitis pigmentosa-36
611131 [39]	NR2E3	Retinitis pigmentosa-37
268000 [3]	MERTK	Retinitis pigmentosa-38
268000 [3]	USH2A	Retinitis pigmentosa-39
612095 [40]	PROM1	Retinitis pigmentosa-41

612943 [41]	KLHL7	Retinitis pigmentosa-42
268000 [3]	CNGB1	Retinitis pigmentosa-45
613194 [42]	BEST1	Retinitis pigmentosa-50
613464 [43]	TTC8	Retinitis pigmentosa 51
613428 [44]	C2orf71	Retinitis pigmentosa 54
613575 [45]	ARL6	Retinitis pigmentosa 55
613617 [46]	ZNF513	Retinitis pigmentosa 58
613194 [42]	BEST1	Retinitis pigmentosa, concentric
608133 [22]	PRPH2	Retinitis pigmentosa, digenic
613341 [47]	LRAT	Retinitis pigmentosa, juvenile
268000 [3]	SPATA7	Retinitis pigmentosa, juvenile, autosomal recessive
268000 [3]	CRX	Retinitis pigmentosa, late-onset dominant
300455 [48]	RPGR	Retinitis pigmentosa, X-linked, and sinorespiratory infections, with or without deafness

The rhodopsin gene encodes a principal protein of photoreceptor outer segments. Studies show that mutations in this gene are responsible for approximately 25% of autosomal dominant forms of RP.[16] [49]

Mutations in four pre-mRNA splicing factors are known to cause autosomal dominant retinitis pigmentosa. These are PRPF3, PRPF8, PRPF31 and PAP1. These factors are ubiquitously expressed and it is still a puzzle as to why defects in a ubiquitous factor should only cause disease in the retina.

Up to 150 mutations have been reported to date in the opsin gene associated with the RP since the Pro23His mutation in the intradiscal domain of the protein was first reported in 1990. These mutations are found throughout the opsin gene and are distributed along the three domains of the protein (the intradiscal, transmembrane, and cytoplasmic domains). One of the main biochemical causes of RP in the case of rhodopsin mutations is protein misfolding, and molecular chaperones have also been involved in RP.[50] It was found that the mutation of codon 23 in the rhodopsin gene, in which proline is changed to histidine, accounts for the largest fraction of rhodopsin mutations in the United States. Several other studies have reported other mutations which also correlate with the disease. These mutations include Thr58Arg, Pro347Leu, Pro347Ser, as well as deletion of Ile-255.[49] [51] [52] [53] [54] In 2000, a rare mutation in codon 23 was reported causing autosomal dominant retinitis pigmentosa, in which proline changed to alanine. However, this study showed that the retinal dystrophy associated with this mutation was characteristically mild in presentation and course. Furthermore, there was greater preservation in electroretinography amplitudes than the more prevalent Pro23His mutation.[55]

Treatment

Although incurable, the progression of the disease can be reduced by the daily intake of 15000 IU (equivalent to 4.5 mg) of vitamin A palmitate.[56] Recent studies have shown that proper vitamin A supplementation can postpone blindness by up to 10 years (by reducing the 10% loss pa to 8.3% pa).[57]

Research on possible treatments

Future treatments may involve retinal transplants, artificial retinal implants,[58] gene therapy, stem cells, nutritional supplements, and/or drug therapies.

2006: Stem cells: UK Researchers working with mice, transplanted mouse stem cells which were at an advanced stage of development, and already programmed to develop into photoreceptor cells, into mice that had been genetically induced to mimic the human conditions of retinitis pigmentosa and age-related macular degeneration. These photoreceptors developed and made the necessary neural connections to the animal's retinal nerve cells, a key step in the restoration of sight. Previously it was believed that the mature retina has no regenerative ability. This research may in the future lead to using transplants in humans to relieve blindness.[59]

2008: Scientists at the Osaka Bioscience Institute have identified a protein, named Pikachurin, which they believe could lead to a treatment for retinitis pigmentosa.[60] [61]

2010: A possible gene therapy seems to work in mice.[5]

2010:R-Tech Ueno(Japanese Medicine manufacture enterprise)Completes Phase II Clinical Study on Ophthalmic Solution UF-021 (Product Name Ocuseva (TM)) on Retinitis Pigmentosa

Notable people with RP

- William Baird, from the New Zealand metal band 'Mëat'
- Willie Brown, former Mayor of San Francisco
- Viviane Forest, Canadian Paralympic alpine skier
- Gordon Gund, U.S. sports team owner
- Sheena Iyengar, Management Guru
- Jim Knipfel, American novelist, autobiographer, and journalist
- Amar Latif Scottish entrepreneur, television actor, director and motivational speaker
- Isaac Lidsky, former child actor and first blind US Supreme Court clerk
- Tony Sarre, Filmmaker
- Woody Shaw, American jazz musician
- Amanda Swafford, American supermodel and television personality
- John Totleben, American illustrator
- Rigo Tovar, Mexican singer, composer, songwriter
- Mildred Weisenfeld, founder of the Fight for Sight eye research foundation in 1946.
- Jon Wellner, actor[62]
- Steve Wynn, Las Vegas casino developer[63]
- Richard Bernstein, lawyer, triathlon athlete, rights advocate for the visually impaired

References

[1] http://apps.who.int/classifications/apps/icd/icd10online/?gh30.htm+h355

[2] http://www.icd9data.com/getICD9Code.ashx?icd9=362.74

[3] http://www.ncbi.nlm.nih.gov/omim/268000

[4] http://www.nlm.nih.gov/cgi/mesh/2010/MB_cgi?field=uid&term=D012174

[5] "Genetic Reactivation of Cone Photoreceptors Restores Visual Responses in Retinitis pigmentosa" (http://www.sciencemag.org/cgi/content/abstract/science.1190897v1). .

[6] Koenekoop, R.K. (2003). Novel RPGR mutations with distinct retinitis pigmentosa phenotypes in French-Canadian families. *American journal of ophthalmology* 136(4), pp. 678-68

[7] http://www.genenames.org/data/hgnc_data.php?match=RLBP1

[8] http://www.genenames.org/data/hgnc_data.php?match=RP1

[9] http://www.genenames.org/data/hgnc_data.php?match=RHO

[10] http://www.genenames.org/data/hgnc_data.php?match=RDS

[11] http://www.genenames.org/data/hgnc_data.php?match=PRPF8

[12] http://www.genenames.org/data/hgnc_data.php?match=PRPF3

[13] http://www.genenames.org/data/hgnc_data.php?match=ABCA4

[14] http://www.genenames.org/data/hgnc_data.php?match=RPE65

[15] http://emedicine.medscape.com/article/1227488-diagnosis

[16] Hartong DT, Berson EL, Dryja TP (November 2006). "Retinitis pigmentosa". *Lancet* **368** (9549): 1795–809. doi:10.1016/S0140-6736(06)69740-7. PMID 17113430.

[17] Farrar GJ, Kenna PF, Humphries P (March 2002). "On the genetics of retinitis pigmentosa and on mutation-independent approaches to therapeutic intervention" (http://www.pubmedcentral.nih.gov/articlerender.fcgi?tool=pmcentrez&artid=125887). *EMBO J.* **21** (5): 857–64. doi:10.1093/emboj/21.5.857. PMID 11867514. PMC 125887.

[18] Online 'Mendelian Inheritance in Man' (OMIM) RETINITIS PIGMENTOSA; RP -268000 (http://www.ncbi.nlm.nih.gov/omim/268000)

[19] http://www.ncbi.nlm.nih.gov/omim/180100

[20] http://www.ncbi.nlm.nih.gov/omim/312600

[21] http://www.ncbi.nlm.nih.gov/omim/300029

[22] http://www.ncbi.nlm.nih.gov/omim/608133

[23] http://www.ncbi.nlm.nih.gov/omim/180104

[24] http://www.ncbi.nlm.nih.gov/omim/180105

[25] http://www.ncbi.nlm.nih.gov/omim/600138

[26] http://www.ncbi.nlm.nih.gov/omim/600105

[27] http://www.ncbi.nlm.nih.gov/omim/600059

[28] http://www.ncbi.nlm.nih.gov/omim/600132

[29] http://www.ncbi.nlm.nih.gov/omim/600852

[30] http://www.ncbi.nlm.nih.gov/omim/601414

[31] http://www.ncbi.nlm.nih.gov/omim/601718

[32] http://www.ncbi.nlm.nih.gov/omim/602772

[33] http://www.ncbi.nlm.nih.gov/omim/608380

[34] http://www.ncbi.nlm.nih.gov/omim/607921

[35] http://www.ncbi.nlm.nih.gov/omim/609923

[36] http://www.ncbi.nlm.nih.gov/omim/610359

[37] http://www.ncbi.nlm.nih.gov/omim/610282

[38] http://www.ncbi.nlm.nih.gov/omim/610599

[39] http://www.ncbi.nlm.nih.gov/omim/611131

[40] http://www.ncbi.nlm.nih.gov/omim/612095

[41] http://www.ncbi.nlm.nih.gov/omim/612943

[42] http://www.ncbi.nlm.nih.gov/omim/613194

[43] http://www.ncbi.nlm.nih.gov/omim/613464

[44] http://www.ncbi.nlm.nih.gov/omim/613428

[45] http://www.ncbi.nlm.nih.gov/omim/613575

[46] http://www.ncbi.nlm.nih.gov/omim/613617

[47] http://www.ncbi.nlm.nih.gov/omim/613341

[48] http://www.ncbi.nlm.nih.gov/omim/300455

[49] Berson EL, Rosner B, Sandberg MA, Dryja TP (January 1991). "Ocular findings in patients with autosomal dominant retinitis pigmentosa and a rhodopsin gene defect (Pro-23-His)". *Arch. Ophthalmol.* **109** (1): 92–101. PMID 1987956.

[50] Senin II, Bosch L, Ramon E, *et al.* (October 2006). "Ca^{2+}/recoverin dependent regulation of phosphorylation of the rhodopsin mutant R135L associated with retinitis pigmentosa". *Biochem. Biophys. Res. Commun.* **349** (1): 345–52. doi:10.1016/j.bbrc.2006.08.048. PMID 16934219.

[51] Dryja TP, McGee TL, Reichel E, *et al.* (January 1990). "A point mutation of the rhodopsin gene in one form of retinitis pigmentosa". *Nature* **343** (6256): 364–6. doi:10.1038/343364a0. PMID 2137202.

[52] Dryja TP, McGee TL, Hahn LB, *et al.* (November 1990). "Mutations within the rhodopsin gene in patients with autosomal dominant retinitis pigmentosa". *N. Engl. J. Med.* **323** (19): 1302–7. doi:10.1056/NEJM199011083231903. PMID 2215617.

[53] Berson EL, Rosner B, Sandberg MA, Weigel-DiFranco C, Dryja TP (May 1991). "Ocular findings in patients with autosomal dominant retinitis pigmentosa and rhodopsin, proline-347-leucine". *Am. J. Ophthalmol.* **111** (5): 614–23. PMID 2021172.

[54] Inglehearn CF, Bashir R, Lester DH, Jay M, Bird AC, Bhattacharya SS (January 1991). "A 3-bp deletion in the rhodopsin gene in a family with autosomal dominant retinitis pigmentosa" (http://www.pubmedcentral.nih.gov/articlerender.fcgi?tool=pmcentrez&artid=1682750). *Am. J. Hum. Genet.* **48** (1): 26–30. PMID 1985460. PMC 1682750.

[55] Oh KT, Weleber RG, Lotery A, Oh DM, Billingslea AM, Stone EM (September 2000). "Description of a new mutation in rhodopsin, Pro23Ala, and comparison with electroretinographic and clinical characteristics of the Pro23His mutation" (http://archopht.ama-assn.org/cgi/pmidlookup?view=long&pmid=10980774). *Arch. Ophthalmol.* **118** (9): 1269–76. PMID 10980774. .

[56] Berson EL, Rosner B, Sandberg MA, *et al.* (1993). "A randomized trial of vitamin A and vitamin E supplementation for retinitis pigmentosa". *Arch. Ophthalmol.* **111** (6): 761–72. PMID 8512476.

[57] Berson EL (2007). "Long-term visual prognoses in patients with retinitis pigmentosa: the Ludwig von Sallmann lecture" (http://www.pubmedcentral.nih.gov/articlerender.fcgi?tool=pmcentrez&artid=2892386). *Exp. Eye Res.* **85** (1): 7–14. doi:10.1016/j.exer.2007.03.001. PMID 17531222. PMC 2892386.

[58] Rush University Medical Center (2005-01-31). "Ophthalmologists Implant Five Patients with Artificial Silicon Retina Microchip To Treat Vision Loss from Retinitis Pigmentosa" (http://www.rush.edu/webapps/MEDREL/servlet/NewsRelease?ID=608). Press release. . Retrieved 2007-06-16.

[59] MacLaren, RE; RA Pearson, A MacNeil, RH Douglas, TE Salt, M Akimoto, A Swaroop, JC Sowden, RR Ali (2006-11-09). "Retinal repair by transplantation of photoreceptor precursors". *Nature* **444** (7116): 203–7. doi:10.1038/nature05161. PMID 17093405.

[60] Sato S, Omori Y, Katoh K, *et al.* (August 2008). "Pikachurin, a dystroglycan ligand, is essential for photoreceptor ribbon synapse formation". *Nat. Neurosci.* **11** (8): 923–931. doi:10.1038/nn.2160. PMID 18641643.

[61] Lightning-Fast Vision Protein Named After Pikachu (http://www.inventorspot.com/articles/lightningfast_vision_protein_named_after_pikachu_16170) July 24, 2008

[62] "CSI Cast: Jon Wellner" (http://www.cbs.com/primetime/csi/cast/jon-wellner/). CBS. . Retrieved October 5, 2010.

[63] http://www.newyorker.com/archive/2006/10/23/061023ta_talk_paumgarten

External links

- Retinitis pigmentosa (http://www.dmoz.org/Health/Conditions_and_Diseases/Eye_Disorders/Retina/Retinitis_Pigmentosa//) at the Open Directory Project

Human eye

This article deals with the human eye, for the description of this organ in other animal, see eye.

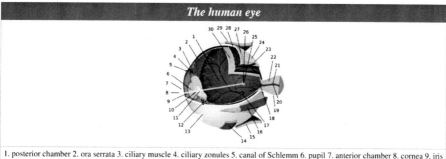

The human eye

1. posterior chamber 2. ora serrata 3. ciliary muscle 4. ciliary zonules 5. canal of Schlemm 6. pupil 7. anterior chamber 8. cornea 9. iris 10. lens cortex 11. lens nucleus 12. ciliary process 13. conjunctiva 14. inferior oblique muscle 15. inferior rectus muscle 16. medial rectus muscle 17. retinal arteries and veins 18. optic disc 19. dura mater 20. central retinal artery 21. central retinal vein 22. optic nerve 23. vorticose vein 24. bulbar sheath 25. macula 26. fovea 27. sclera 28. choroid 29. superior rectus muscle 30. retina

The **human eye** is an organ which reacts to light for several purposes.

As a conscious sense organ, the eye allows vision. Rod and cone cells in the retina allow conscious light perception and vision including color differentiation and the perception of depth. The human eye can distinguish about 10 million colors.[1]

In common with the eyes of other mammals, the human eye's non-image-forming photosensitive ganglion cells in the retina receive the light signals which affect adjustment of the size of the pupil, regulation and suppression of the hormone melatonin and entrainment of the body clock.

General properties

The eye is not properly a sphere, rather it is a fused two-piece unit. The smaller frontal unit, more curved, called the cornea is linked to the larger unit called the sclera. The corneal segment is typically about 8 mm (0.3 in) in radius. The sclera constitutes the remaining five-sixths; its radius is typically about 12 mm. The cornea and sclera are connected by a ring called the limbus. The iris – the color of the eye – and its black center, the pupil, are seen instead of the cornea due to the cornea's transparency. To see inside the eye, an ophthalmoscope is needed, since light is not reflected out. The fundus (area opposite the pupil) shows the characteristic pale optic disk (papilla), where vessels entering the eye pass across and optic nerve fibers depart the globe.

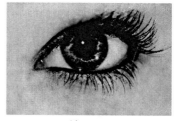

A human eye.

Dimensions

The dimensions differ among adults by only one or two millimeters. The vertical measure, generally less than the horizontal distance, is about 24 mm among adults, at birth about 16–17 mm. (about 0.65 inch) The eyeball grows rapidly, increasing to 22.5–23 mm (approx. 0.89 in) by the age of three years. From then to age 13, the eye attains its full size. The volume is 6.5 ml (0.4 cu. in.) and the weight is 7.5 g. (0.25 oz.)

Components

The eye is made up of three coats, enclosing three transparent structures. The outermost layer is composed of the cornea and sclera. The middle layer consists of the choroid, ciliary body, and iris. The innermost is the retina, which gets its circulation from the vessels of the choroid as well as the retinal vessels, which can be seen in an ophthalmoscope.

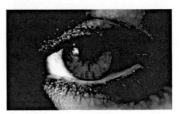

A woman's eye.

Within these coats are the aqueous humor, the vitreous body, and the flexible lens. The aqueous humor is a clear fluid that is contained in two areas: the anterior chamber between the cornea and the iris and exposed area of the lens; and the posterior chamber, behind the iris and the rest. The lens is suspended to the ciliary body by the suspensory ligament (Zonule of Zinn), made up of fine transparent fibers. The vitreous body is a clear jelly that is much larger than the aqueous humor, and is bordered by the sclera, zonule, and lens. They are connected via the pupil.[2]

Dynamic range

The retina has a static contrast ratio of around 100:1 (about 6½ f-stops). As soon as the eye moves (saccades) it re-adjusts its exposure both chemically and geometrically by adjusting the iris which regulates the size of the pupil. Initial dark adaptation takes place in approximately four seconds of profound, uninterrupted darkness; full adaptation through adjustments in retinal chemistry (the Purkinje effect) are mostly complete in thirty minutes. Hence, a dynamic contrast ratio of about 1,000,000:1 (about 20 f-stops) is possible.[3] The process is nonlinear and multifaceted, so an interruption by light merely starts the adaptation process over again. Full adaptation is dependent on good blood flow; thus dark adaptation may be hampered by poor circulation, and vasoconstrictors like alcohol or tobacco.

The eye includes a lens not dissimilar to lenses found in optical instruments such as cameras and the same principles can be applied. The pupil of the human eye is its aperture; the iris is the diaphragm that serves as the aperture stop. Refraction in the cornea causes the effective aperture (the entrance pupil) to differ slightly from the physical pupil diameter. The entrance pupil is typically about 4 mm in diameter, although it can range from 2 mm (f/8.3) in a brightly lit place to 8 mm (f/2.1) in the dark. The latter value decreases slowly with age, older people's eyes sometimes dilate to not more than 5-6mm.

Field of view

The approximate field of view of a human eye is 95° out, 75° down, 60° in, 60° up. About 12–15° temporal and 1.5° below the horizontal is the optic nerve or blind spot which is roughly 7.5° high and 5.5° wide.[4]

Eye irritation

Eye irritation has been defined as "the magnitude of any stinging, scratching, burning, or other irritating sensation from the eye".[5] It is a common problem experienced by people of all ages. Related eye symptoms and signs of irritation are e.g. discomfort, dryness, excess tearing, itching, grating, sandy sensation, smarting, ocular fatigue, pain, scratchiness, soreness, redness, swollen eyelids, and tiredness, etc. These eye symptoms are reported with intensities from severe to less severe. It has been suggested that these eye symptoms are related to different causal mechanisms.[6]

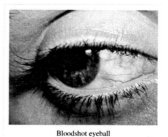
Bloodshot eyeball

Several suspected causal factors in our environment have been studied so far.[7] One hypothesis is that indoor air pollution may cause eye and airway irritation.[8] [9] Eye irritation depends somewhat on destabilization of the outer-eye tear film, in which the formation of dry spots results in such ocular discomfort as dryness.[8] [10] [11] Occupational factors are also likely to influence the perception of eye irritation. Some of these are lighting (glare and poor contrast), gaze position, a limited number of breaks, and a constant function of accommodation, musculoskeletal burden, and impairment of the visual nervous system.[12] [13] Another factor that may be related is work stress.[14] [15] In addition, psychological factors have been found in multivariate analyses to be associated with an increase in eye irritation among VDU users.[16] [17] Other risk factors, such as chemical toxins/irritants, e.g. Amines, Formaldehyde, Acetaldehyde, Acrolein, N-decane, VOCs; Ozone, Pesticides and preservatives, Allergens, etc might cause eye irritation as well.

Certain volatile organic compounds that are both chemically reactive and airway irritants may cause eye irritation as well. Personal factors (e.g., use of contact lenses, eye make-up, and certain medications) may also affect destabilization of the tear film and possibly result in more eye symptoms.[6] Nevertheless, if airborne particles alone should destabilize the tear film and cause eye irritation, their content of surface-active compounds must be high.[6] An integrated physiological risk model with blink frequency, destabilization, and break-up of the eye tear film as inseparable phenomena may explain eye irritation among office workers in terms of occupational, climate, and eye-related physiological risk factors.[6]

There are two major measures of eye irritation. One is blink frequency which can be observed by human behavior. The other measures are break up time, tear flow, hyperemia (redness, swelling), tear fluid cytology, and epithelial damage (vital stains) etc, which are human beings' physiological reactions. Blink frequency is defined as the number of blinks per minute and it is associated with eye irritation. Blink frequencies are individual with mean frequencies of < 2-3 to 20-30 blinks/minute, and they depend on environmental factors including the use of contact lenses. Dehydration, mental activities, work conditions, room temperature, relative humidity, and illumination all influence blink frequency. Break-up time (BUT) is another major measure of eye irritation and tear film stability.[18] It is defined as the time interval (in seconds) between blinking and rupture. BUT is considered to reflect the stability of the tear film as well. In normal persons, the break-up time exceeds the interval between blinks, and, therefore, the tear film is maintained.[19] Studies have shown that blink frequency is correlated negatively with break-up time. This phenomenon indicates that perceived eye irritation is associated with an increase in blink frequency since the cornea and conjunctiva both have sensitive nerve endings that belong to the first trigeminal branch.[20] [21] Other evaluating methods, such as hyperemia, cytology etc have increasingly been used to assess eye irritation.

There are other factors that related to eye irritation as well. Three major factors that influence the most are indoor air pollution, contact lenses and gender differences. Field studies have found that the prevalence of objective eye signs is often significantly altered among office workers in comparisons with random samples of the general population.[22] [23] [24] [25] These research results might indicate that indoor air pollution has played an important role in causing eye irritation. There are more and more people wearing contact lens now and dry eyes appear to be the most common complaint among contact lens wearers.[26] [27] [28] Although both contact lens wearers and spectacle wearers experience similar eye irritation symptoms, dryness, redness, and grittiness have been reported far more frequently among contact lens wearers and with greater severity than among spectacle wearers.[28] Studies have shown that incidence of dry eyes increases with age.[29] [30] especially among women. [31] Tear film stability (eg. break-up time) is significantly lower among women than among men. In addition, women have a higher blink frequency while reading.[32] Several factors may contribute to gender differences. One is the use of eye make-up. Another reason could be that the women in the reported studies have done more VDU work than the men, including lower grade work. A third often-quoted explanation is related to the age-dependent decrease of tear secretion, particularly among women after 40 years of age.[33] [34] , [35]

In a study conducted by UCLA, the frequency of reported symptoms in industrial buildings was investigated.[36] The study's results were that eye irritation was the most frequent symptom in industrial building spaces, at 81%. Modern office work with use of office equipment has raised concerns about possible adverse health effects.[37] Since the 1970s, reports have linked mucosal, skin, and general symptoms to work with self-copying paper. Emission of various particulate and volatile substances has been suggested as specific causes. These symptoms have been related to Sick Building Syndrome (SBS), which involves symptoms such as irritation to the eyes, skin, and upper airways, headache and fatigue.[38]

Many of the symptoms described in SBS and multiple chemical sensitivity (MCS) resemble the symptoms known to be elicited by airborne irritant chemicals.[39] A repeated measurement design was employed in the study of acute symptoms of eye and respiratory tract irritation resulting from occupational exposure to sodium borate dusts.[40] The symptom assessment of the 79 exposed and 27 unexposed subjects comprised interviews before the shift began and then at regular hourly intervals for the next six hours of the shift, four days in a row.[40] Exposures were monitored concurrently with a personal real time aerosol monitor. Two different exposure profiles, a daily average and short term (15 minute) average, were used in the analysis. Exposure-response relations were evaluated by linking incidence rates for each symptom with categories of exposure.[40]

Acute incidence rates for nasal, eye, and throat irritation, and coughing and breathlessness were found to be associated with increased exposure levels of both exposure indices. Steeper exposure-response slopes were seen when short term exposure concentrations were used. Results from multivariate logistic regression analysis suggest that current smokers tended to be less sensitive to the exposure to airborne sodium borate dust.[40]

Several actions can be taken to prevent eye irritation—

- trying to maintain normal blinking by avoiding room temperatures that are too high; avoiding relative humidities that are too high or too low, because they reduce blink frequency or may increase water evaporation[6]
- trying to maintain an intact tear film by the following actions. 1) blinking and short breaks may be beneficial for VDU users.[41] [42] Increase these two actions might help maintain the tear film. 2) downward gazing is recommended to reduce the ocular surface area and water evaporation.[43] [44] [45] 3) the distance between the VDU and keyboard should be kept as short as possible to minimize evaporation from the ocular surface area by a low direction of the gaze.[46] And 4) blink training can be beneficial.[47]

In addition, other measures are proper lid hygiene, avoidance of eye rubbing,[48] and proper use of personal products and medication. Eye make-up should be used with care.[49]

Eye movement

The visual system in the brain is too slow to process information if the images are slipping across the retina at more than a few degrees per second.[50] Thus, for humans to be able to see while moving, the brain must compensate for the motion of the head by turning the eyes. Another complication for vision in frontal-eyed animals is the development of a small area of the retina with a very high visual acuity. This area is called the fovea, and covers about 2 degrees of visual angle in people. To get a clear view of the world, the brain must turn the eyes so that the image of the object of regard falls on the fovea. Eye movements are thus very important for visual perception, and any failure to make them correctly can lead to serious visual disabilities.

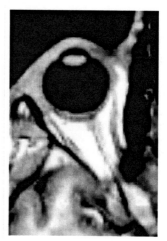

MRI scan of human eye

Having two eyes is an added complication, because the brain must point both of them accurately enough that the object of regard falls on corresponding points of the two retinas; otherwise, double vision would occur. The movements of different body parts are controlled by striated muscles acting around joints. The movements of the eye are no exception, but they have special advantages not shared by skeletal muscles and joints, and so are considerably different.

Extraocular muscles

Each eye has six muscles that control its movements: the lateral rectus, the medial rectus, the inferior rectus, the superior rectus, the inferior oblique, and the superior oblique. When the muscles exert different tensions, a torque is exerted on the globe that causes it to turn, in almost pure rotation, with only about one millimeter of translation.[51] Thus, the eye can be considered as undergoing rotations about a single point in the center of the eye.

Rapid eye movement

Rapid eye movement, or REM for short, typically refers to the sleep stage during which the most vivid dreams occur. During this stage, the eyes move rapidly. It is not in itself a unique form of eye movement.

Saccades

Saccades are quick, simultaneous movements of both eyes in the same direction controlled by the frontal lobe of the brain. Some irregular drifts, movements, smaller than a saccade and larger than a microsaccade, subtend up to six minutes of arc.

Microsaccades

Even when looking intently at a single spot, the eyes drift around. This ensures that individual photosensitive cells are continually stimulated in different degrees. Without changing input, these cells would otherwise stop generating output. Microsaccades move the eye no more than a total of 0.2° in adult humans.

Vestibulo-ocular reflex

The vestibulo-ocular reflex is a reflex eye movement that stabilizes images on the retina during head movement by producing an eye movement in the direction opposite to head movement, thus preserving the image on the center of the visual field. For example, when the head moves to the right, the eyes move to the left, and vice versa.

Smooth pursuit movement

The eyes can also follow a moving object around. This tracking is less accurate than the vestibulo-ocular reflex, as it requires the brain to process incoming visual information and supply feedback. Following an object moving at constant speed is relatively easy, though the eyes will often make saccadic jerks to keep up. The smooth pursuit movement can move the eye at up to 100°/s in adult humans.

It is more difficult to visually estimate speed in low light conditions or while moving, unless there is another point of reference for determining speed.

Optokinetic reflex

The optokinetic reflex is a combination of a saccade and smooth pursuit movement. When, for example, looking out of the window at a moving train, the eyes can focus on a 'moving' train for a short moment (through smooth pursuit), until the train moves out of the field of vision. At this point, the optokinetic reflex kicks in, and moves the eye back to the point where it first saw the train (through a saccade).

Near Response

The adjustment to close-range vision involves three processes to focus an image on the retina.

Vergence movement

When a creature with binocular vision looks at an object, the eyes must rotate around a vertical axis so that the projection of the image is in the centre of the retina in both eyes. To look at an object closer by, the eyes rotate 'towards each other' (convergence), while for an object farther away they rotate 'away from each other' (divergence). Exaggerated convergence is called *cross eyed viewing* (focusing on the nose for example). When looking into the distance, or when 'staring into nothingness', the eyes neither converge nor diverge.

Vergence movements are closely connected to accommodation of the eye. Under normal conditions, changing the focus of the eyes to look at an object at a different distance will automatically cause vergence and accommodation.

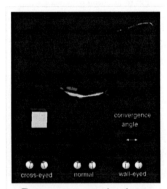

The two eyes converge to point to the same object.

Pupil Constriction

Lenses cannot refract light rays at their edges as well as they can closer to the center. The image produced by any lens is therefore somewhat blurry around the edges (spherical aberration). It can be minimized by screening out peripheral light rays and looking only at the better-focused center. In the eye, the pupil serves this purpose by constricting while the eye is focused on nearby objects. In this way the pupil has a dual purpose: to adjust the eye to variations in brightness and to reduce spherical aberration. [52]

Accommodation of the Lens

A change in the curvature of the lens, accommodation is carried out by the ciliary muscles surrounding the lens contracting. This narrows the diameter of the ciliary body, relaxes the fibers of the suspernsory ligament, and allows the lens to relax into a more convex shape. A more convex lens refracts light more strongly and focuses divergent light rays onto the retina allowing for closer objects to be brought into focus. [53]

Effects of Aging

There are many diseases, disorders, and age-related changes that may affect the eyes and surrounding structures.

As the eye ages certain changes occur that can be attributed solely to the aging process. Most of these anatomic and physiologic processes follow a gradual decline. With aging, the quality of vision worsens due to reasons independent of diseases of the aging eye. While there are many changes of significance in the nondiseased eye, the most functionally important changes seem to be a reduction in pupil size and the loss of accommodation or focusing capability (presbyopia). The area of the pupil governs the amount of light that can reach the retina. The extent to which the pupil dilates decreases with age, leading to a substantial decrease in light received at the retina. In comparison to younger people, it is as though older persons are constantly wearing medium-density sunglasses. Therefore, for any detailed visually guided tasks on which performance varies with illumination, older persons require extra lighting. Certain ocular diseases can come from sexually transmitted diseases such as herpes and genital warts. If contact between eye and area of infection occurs, the STD can be transmitted to the eye.[54]

With aging a prominent white ring develops in the periphery of the cornea- called arcus senilis. Aging causes laxity and downward shift of eyelid tissues and atrophy of the orbital fat. These changes contribute to the etiology of several eyelid disorders such as ectropion, entropion, dermatochalasis, and ptosis. The vitreous gel undergoes liquefaction (posterior vitreous detachment or PVD) and its opacities — visible as floaters — gradually increase in number.

Various eye care professionals, including ophthalmologists, optometrists, and opticians, are involved in the treatment and management of ocular and vision disorders. A Snellen chart is one type of eye chart used to measure visual acuity. At the conclusion of an eye examination, an eye doctor may provide the patient with an eyeglass prescription for corrective lenses. Some disorders of the eyes for which corrective lenses are prescribed include myopia (near-sightedness) which affects one-third of the population, hyperopia (far-sightedness) which affects one quarter of the population, and presbyopia, a loss of focusing range due to aging.

References

[1] Judd, Deane B.; Wyszecki, Günter (1975). *Color in Business, Science and Industry*. Wiley Series in Pure and Applied Optics (third edition ed.). New York: Wiley-Interscience. p. 388. ISBN 0471452122.

[2] "eye, human."Encyclopædia Britannica from Encyclopædia Britannica 2006 Ultimate Reference Suite DVD 2009

[3] Barton, H. and Byrne, K. *Introduction to Human Vision, Visual Defects & Eye Tests* (March 2007), p. 22. PDF (http://opticonsultinguk.com/downloads/Hugh_Barton-Kerry_Byrne_20070330.pdf)

[4] MIL-STD-1472F, Military Standard, Human Engineering, Design Criteria For Military Systems, Equipment, And Facilities (23 Aug 1999) PDF (http://www.everyspec.com/MIL-STD/MIL-STD+(1400+-+1499)/download.php?spec=MIL_STD_1472F.1208.pdf)

[5] Mendell MJ. Non-specific symptoms in office workers: a review and summary of the epidemiologic literature. Indoor Air 1993; 3: 227-36.

[6] Wolkoff, P., Skov, P., Franck, C., and Petersen, LN. "Eye irritation and environmental factors in the office environment-hypotheses, causes and a physiological model" Scandinavian Journal of Work, Environment & Health [Scand. J. Work Environ. Health]. Dec 2003, pp. 411–430. Vol. 29, No. 6.

[7] Mendell MJ. Non-specific symptoms in office workers: a review and summary of the epidemiologic literature. Indoor Air 1993; 3: 227-36

[8] Norn MS. Pollution keratoconjunctivitis. Acta Ophthalmol Scand 1992; 70: 269-73.

[9] Versura P, Profazio V, Cellini M, Torreggiani A, Caramazza R. Eye discomfort and air pollution. Ophthalmologica 1999; 213: 103-9

[10] Lemp MA. New strategies in the treatment of dry-eye states. Cornea 1999; 18: 625-32.

[11] Rolando M, Zierhurt M. The ocular surface and tear film and their dysfuction in dry eye disease. Surv Ophthalmol 2001; 45: S203-S210

[12] Murata K, Araki S, Kawakami N, Saito Y, Hino E. Central nervous system effects and visual fatigue in VDT workers. Int Arch Occup Health 1991; 63: 109-13

[13] Rossignol AM, Morse EP, Summers VM, Pagnotto LD. Video display terminal use and reported health symptoms among Massachusetts clerical workers. J Occup Med 1987; 29: 112-8

[14] Apter A, Bracker A, Hodgson M, Sidman J, Leung W-Y. Epidemiology of the sick building syndrome. J Allergy Clin Immunol 1994; 94: 277-88.

[15] Thomas WD. Eye problems and visual display terminals- the facts and the fallacies. Opthalmic Physiol Opt 2001; 18: 111-9

[16] Aronsson G, Stromberg A. Work content and eye discomfort in VDT work. Int J Occup Saf Ergon 1995; 1: 1-13

[17] Mocci F, Serra A, Corrias GA. Psychological factors and visual fatigue in working with video display terminals. Occup Environ Med 2001; 58: 267-71

[18] Kjaergaard, SK. Chapter 17. The irritated eye in the indoor environment, Indoor Air Quality Handbook

[19] Wolkoff, P., Skov, P., Franck, C., and Petersen, LN. "Eye irritation and environmental factors in the office environment-hypotheses, causes and a physiological model" Scandinavian Journal of Work, Environment & Health. Dec 2003, pp. 411-430, Vol. 29, No.6

[20] Norn Ms. External eye: methods of examination. Copenhagen: Scriptor; 1983

[21] Sibony PA, Evinger C. Anatomy and physiology of normal and abnormal eyelid position and movement. In: Miller NR, Newman NJ, editors. Walsh & Hoyt's clinical neuro-ophthalmology. Baltimore (MD): Williams and Wilkins; 1998. P 1509- 92

[22] Franck C, Back E, Skov P. Prevalence of objective eye manifestations in people working in office buildings with different prevalence of the sick building syndrome compared with the general population. Int Arch Occup Health 1993; 65: 65- 9

[23] Franck C. Fatty layer of the precorneal film in the 'office eye syndrome'. Acta Ophthalmol Scand 1991; 69: 737- 43

[24] Franck C, Skov P. Foam at inner eye canthus in office workers, compared with an average Danish population as control group. Acta Ophthalmol Scand 1989; 67: 61- 8

[25] Franck C. Eye symptoms and signs in buildings with indoor climate problems ('Office Eye Syndroms'). Acta Ophthalmol Scand 1986; 64: 306- 11

[26] Doughty MJ, Fonn D, Richter D, Simpson T, Caffery B, Gordon K. A patient questionnaire approach to estimating the prevalence of dry eye symptoms in patients presenting to optometric practices across Canada. Optom Vis Sci 1997; 74: 424- 31.

[27] Fonn D, Situ P, Simpsom T. Hydrogel lens dehydration and subjective comfort and dryness Ratings in symptomatic and asymptomatic contact lens wearers. Optom Vis Sci 1999; 76: 700- 4

[28] Vajdic C, Holden BA, Sweeney DF, Cornish RM. The frequency of ocular symptoms during spectacle and daily soft and rigid contact lens wear. Optom Vis Sci 1999; 76: 705- 11

[29] Seal, D. V., and I. A. Mackie. 1986. The questionable dry eye as a clinical and biochemical entity. In F. J. Holly (Ed.), the preocular tear film – In health, disease, and contact lens wear. Dry Eye Institute, Lubbock, Texas, 41- 51

[30] Hikichi, T., A. Yoshida, Y. Fukui, T. Hamano, M. Ri, K. Araki, K. Horimoto, E. Takamura, K. Kitagawa, M. Oyama, Y. Danjo, S. Kondo, H. Fujishima, I. Toda, and K. Tsubota. 1995. Prevalence of dry eye in Japanese eye centers. Graefe's Arch. Clin. Exp. Ophthalmol. 233: 555-558.

[31] McCarty, C. A., A. K. Bansal, P. M. Livingston, Y. L. Stanislovsky, and H. R. Taylor. 1998. The Epidemiology of Dry Eye in Melbourne, Australia. Ophthalmology 105: 1114- 1119

[32] Bentivoglio AR, Bressman SB, Cassetta E. Caretta D, Tonali P, Albanese A. Analysis of blink rate patterns in normal subjects. Mov Disord 1997; 1028- 34

[33] McCarty CA, Bansal AK, Livingston PM, Stanislavsky YL, Taylor HR. The epidemiology of dry eye in Melbourne, Australia. Ophthalmology 1998; 105: 1114- 9

[34] Mathers WD, Lane JA, Zimmerman MB. Tear film changes associated with normal aging. Cornea 1996; 15: 229- 34

[35] Mathers WD, Stovall D, Lane JA, Zimmerman MB, Johnson S. Menopause and tear function: the influence of prolactin and sex hormones on human tear production. Cornea 1998; 17: 353- 8

[36] Wallingford K.M and Carpenter, J Proc. IAQ '86: Managing Indoor Air for Health and Energy Conserv., American Society for Heating, Refrigerating, and Air-Conditioning Engineers, Atlanta, 448, 1986.

[37] Jaakkola, Maritta S. and Jouni J. K. Jaakkola. "Office Equipment and Supplies: A Modern Occupational Health Concern?", American Journal of Epidemiology, 1999, pp. 1223, Vol. 150, No. 11

[38] Nordström K., D. Norbäck, and R. Akselsson. "Influence of indoor air quality and personal factors on the sick building syndrome (SBS) in Swedish geriatric hospitals.", Occupational and Environmental Medicine, 1995, pp. 170–176, Vol. 52.

[39] Anderson, Crosalind C. and Julius H. Anderson. "Sensory irritation and multiple chemical sensitivity." Toxicology and Industrial Health, 1999, pp. 339–345, Vol. 15, No. 3-4

[40] X Hu, D H Wegman, E A Eisen, S R Woskie and R G Smith. "Dose related acute irritant symptom responses to occupational exposure to sodium borate dusts." British Journal of Industrial Medicine 1992, pp. 706–713, Vol. 49.

[41] Carney LG, Hill RM. The nature of normal blinking patterns. Acta Ophthalmol Scand 1982; 60: 427- 33

[42] Henning RA, Jacques P, Kissel GV, Sullivan AB, Alteras-Webb SM. Frequent short rest breaks from computer work: effects on productivity and well-being at two field sites. Ergonomics 1997; 40: 78- 91

[43] Nakamori K, Odawara M, Nakajima K, Mizutani T, Tsubota K. Blinking is controlled primarily by ocular surface conditions. Am Ophthalmol 1997; 124: 24-30.

[44] Barbato G, Ficca G, Muscettola G, Fichele M, Beatrice M, Rinaldi F. Diurnal variation in spontaneous eye-blink rate. Psychiatry Res 2000; 93: 145-51.

[45] Sotoyama M, Villanuveva MBG, Jonai H, Saito S. Ocular surface area as an informative index of visual ergonomics. Ind Health 1995; 33: 43- 56

[46] Sotoyama M, Jonai H, Saito S, Villanuveva MBG. Analysis of ocular surface area for comfortable VDT workstation layout. Ergonomics 1996; 39: 877- 84

[47] Collins M, Heron H, Larsen R, Lindner R. Blinking patterns in soft contact lens wearers can be altered with training. Am J Optometry Physiolog Opt 1987; 64: 100-3

[48] Piccoli B, Assini R, Gambaro S, Pastoni F, D'Orso M, Franceshini S, et al. Microbiological pollution and ocular infection in CAS operators: an on-site investigation. Ergonomics 2001; 44: 658- 67

[49] Lozato PA, Pisella PJ, Baudoin C. The lipid layer of the lacrimal tear film: physiology and pathology. J Fr Ophthalmol 2001; 24: 643- 58

[50] Westheimer, Gerald & McKee, Suzanne P.; "Visual acuity in the presence of retinal-image motion". *Journal of the Optical Society of America* 1975 **65**(7), 847–50.

[51] Roger H.S. Carpenter (1988); *Movements of the eyes (2nd ed.)*. Pion Ltd, London. ISBN 0-85086-109-8.

[52] Saladin, Kenneth S. Anatomy and Phyisology: The Unity of Form and Function. 5th ed. New York: McGraw-Hill, 2010. 620–22.

[53] "human eye." Encyclopædia Britannica. 2010. Encyclopædia Britannica Online. 05 Dec. 2010 <http://www.britannica.com/EBchecked/topic/1688997/human-eye>.

[54] AgingEye Times (http://www.agingeye.net/)

External links

- 🔊 Media related to human eyes at Wikimedia Commons

zh-hk:人眼

Nyctalopia

Nyctalopia	
Classification and external resources	
ICD-10	H 53.6 [1]
ICD-9	368.6 [2]

Nyctalopia (from Greek νύκτ-, *nykt-* "night"; and αλαός, *alaos* "blindness") is a condition making it difficult or impossible to see in relatively low light. It is a symptom of several eye diseases. Night blindness may exist from birth, or be caused by injury or malnutrition (for example, a lack of vitamin A). It can be described as insufficient adaptation to darkness.

The most common cause of nyctalopia is retinitis pigmentosa, a disorder in which the rod cells in the retina gradually lose their ability to respond to the light. Patients suffering from this genetic condition have progressive nyctalopia and eventually their daytime vision may also be affected. In X-linked congenital stationary night blindness, from birth the rods either do not work at all, or work very little, but the condition doesn't get worse. Another cause of night blindness is a deficiency of retinol, or vitamin A, found in fish oils, liver and dairy products. In the Second World War disinformation was used by the British to cover up the reason for their pilots' successful nighttime missions. Their success was, in the disinformation, attributed to improved night vision and pilots flying night missions were encouraged to eat plenty of carrots, which contain carotenoids and can be converted into retinol. The real reason for their success was their use of advanced radar technologies.

The opposite problem, the inability to see in bright light, is known as *hemeralopia* and is much rarer.

The outer area of the retina is made up of more rods than cones. The rod cells are the cells that enable us to see in poor illumination. This is the reason why loss of side vision often results in night blindness. Individuals suffering from night blindness not only see poorly at night, but also require some time for their eyes to adjust from brightly lit areas to dim ones. Contrast vision may also be greatly reduced.

Refractive "vision correction" surgery is a widespread cause of nyctalopia due to the impairment of contrast sensitivity function (CSF) which is induced by intraocular light-scatter resulting from surgical intervention in the natural structural integrity of the cornea.[3]

Night blindness is much more common among men than women.

Causes

- Vitamin A deficiency
- retinitis pigmentosa
- congenital night blindness
- Sorsby's fundus dystrophy
- pathological myopia
- peripheral cortical cataract
- oguchi disease
- refractive surgery (RK, PRK, LASIK)

Historical usage

Aulus Cornelius Celsus, writing ca. 30 AD, described night blindness and recommended an effective dietary supplement: "There is besides a weakness of the eyes, owing to which people see well enough indeed in the daytime but not at all at night; in women whose menstruation is regular this does not happen. But success sufferers should anoint their eyeballs with the stuff dripping from a liver whilst roasting, preferably of a he-goat, or failing that of a she-goat; and as well they should eat some of the liver itself."

Historically, nyctalopia, also known as **moonblink**, was a temporary night blindness believed to be caused by sleeping in moonlight in the tropics.[4]

Nyctalopia with animals

Congenital stationary night blindness is also an opthalmologic disorder in horses with leopard spotting patterns, such as the Appaloosa. It is present at birth (congenital), not sex-linked, non-progressive and affects the animal's vision in conditions of low lighting.[5] CSNB is usually diagnosed based on the owner's observations, but some horses have visibly abnormal eyes: poorly-aligned eyes (dorsomedial strabismus) or involuntary eye movement (nystagmus).[5] In horses, CSNB s has been linked with the leopard complex color pattern since the 1970s.[6] A 2008 study theorizes that both CSNB and leopard complex spotting patterns are linked to the TRPM1 gene.[7] The gene to which *Lp* has now been localized encodes a protein that channels calcium ions, a key factor in the transmission of nerve impulses. This protein, which is found in the retina and the skin, existed in fractional percentages of the normal levels in homozygous *Lp/Lp* horses.[5]

References

[1]   http://apps.who.int/classifications/apps/icd/icd10online/?gh53.htm+h536

[2]   http://www.icd9data.com/getICD9Code.ashx?icd9=368.6

[3]   Laser in situ keratomileusis for myopia and the contrast sensitivity function Nadia-Marie Quesnel, John V Lovasik, Christian Ferremi, Martin Boileau, Catherine Ieraci Journal of Cataract & Refractive Surgery June 2004 (Vol. 30, Issue 6, Pages 1209-1218)

[4]   *The Sailor's Word-Book*, Admiral W.H. Smyth, p. 483; Conway Maritime Press, UK, 1991. ISBN 0-85177-972-7

[5]   Bellone, Rebecca R; Brooks SA, Sandmeyer L, Murphy BA, Forsyth G, Archer S, Bailey E, Grahn B (August 2008). "Differential Gene Expression of TRPM1, the Potential Cause of Congenital Stationary Night Blindness and Coat Spotting Patterns (LP) in the Appaloosa Horse (Equus caballus)" (http://www.pubmedcentral.nih.gov/articlerender.fcgi?tool=pmcentrez&artid=2516064). *Genetics* (Genetics Society of America) **179** (179): 1861–1870. doi:10.1534/genetics.108.088807. PMID 18660533. PMC 2516064.

[6]   Witzel CA, Joyce JR, Smith EL. *Electroretinography of congenital night blindness in an Appaloosa filly.* Journal of Equine Medicine and Surgery 1977; 1: 226–229.

[7]   Oke, Stacey, DVM, MSc (August 31, 2008). "Shedding Light on Night Blindness in Appaloosas" (http://www.thehorse.com/ViewArticle. aspx?ID=12595) (Registration required). *The Horse.* . Retrieved 2009-02-07.

Tunnel vision

Tunnel vision (also called "Kalnienk Vision") is the loss of peripheral vision with retention of central vision, resulting in a constricted circular tunnel-like field of vision.[1]

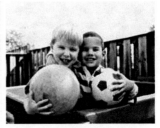

Normal vision. Courtesy NIH National Eye Institute.

Medical / biological causes

Tunnel vision can be caused by:

- Blood loss (hypovolemia)
- Alcohol consumption causes tunnel vision [2]. In addition, the vision becomes blurred or double since eye muscles lose their precision causing them to be unable to focus on the same object.
- Retinitis pigmentosa, a disease of the eye.
- Sustained (1 second or more) high accelerations[3]. Typically, flying an airplane with a centripetal acceleration of up to or over 39 m/s^2 (4gs) with the head towards the center of curvature, common in aerobatic or fighter pilots. In these cases, tunnel vision and greyout may proceed to or g-force induced Loss Of Consciousness (g-LOC).
- Hallucinogenic drugs, in particular the Dissociatives.
- Glaucoma, a disease of the eye.
- Extreme fear or distress, most often in the context of a panic attack.
- During periods of high adrenaline production, such as an intense physical fight.

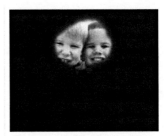

The same view with tunnel vision from retinitis pigmentosa.

- Altitude sickness, hypoxia in passenger aircraft[4]
- Exposure to oxygen at a partial pressure above 1.5-2 atmospheres, producing central nervous system oxygen toxicity, notably while diving.[5] Other symptoms can include dizziness, nausea, blindness, fatigue, anxiety, confusion and lack of coordination.
- Other loss of blood to the brain.
- Prolonged exposure to air contaminated with heated hydraulic fluids and oils, as can sometimes happen in passenger aircraft[6].
- Pituitary stalk mass (i.e. tumor) compressing the optic chiasm
- Severe cataracts, causing a removal of most of the field of vision
- During the aura phase of a migraine
- Intense anger, due to the body being rapidly flooded with adrenaline and oxygen
- A bite from a Black Mamba and other snakes with the same strength venom.

When combined with piloting an aircraft, driving, crossing roads or operating heavy machinery, the consequences can be fatal.

Eyeglass users

Eyeglass users experience tunnel vision to varying degrees due to the corrective lens only providing a small area of proper focus, with the rest of the field of view beyond the lenses being unfocused and blurry.

Where a naturally sighted person only needs to move their eyes to see an object far to the side or far down, the eyeglass wearer may need to move their whole skull to point the eyeglasses towards the target object.

The eyeglass frame also blocks the view of the world with a thin opaque boundary separating the lens area from the rest of the field of view. The eyeglass frame is capable of obscuring small objects and details in the peripheral field.

Mask, goggle, and helmet users

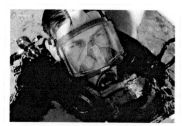
Wide-field, wrap-around diving mask.

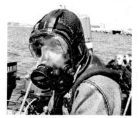
Diving mask with narrow field of view.

Activities which require a protective mask, safety goggles, or fully enclosing protective helmet can also result in an experience approximating tunnel vision.

Underwater diving masks using a single flat transparent lens usually have the lens surface several centimeters from the eyes. The lens is typically enclosed with an opaque black rubber sealing shell to keep out water. For this type of mask the peripheral field of the diver is extremely limited. Generally, the peripheral field of a diving mask is improved if the lenses are as close to the eye as possible, or if the lenses are large, multi-window, or is a curved wrap-around design.

Protective helmets such as a welding helmet restrict vision to an extremely small slot or hole, with no peripheral perception at all. This is done out of necessity so that ultraviolet radiation emitted from the welding arc does not damage the welder's eyes due to reflections off of shiny objects in the peripheral field.

Optical instruments

Binoculars, telescopes, and microscopes induce an experience of extreme tunnel vision due to the design of the optical components.

A wide field microscope or telescope generally requires much larger diameter and thicker lenses, or complex parabolic mirror assemblies, either of which results in significantly greater cost for construction of the optical device.

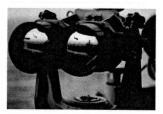
Extremely large wide-field binoculars that would be impractical to carry.

Wide-field binoculars are possible, but the far end lenses would have to be several centimeters in diameter to widen the field of view, resulting in a bulky device that is difficult to transport and store.

References

[1] Medical terms (http://www.medterms.com/script/main/art.asp?articlekey=24514)

[2] Effects of Alcohol on Vision (http://www.cs.wright.edu/bie/rehabengr/vision/visionalcohol.htm)

[3] Web Archive: Virtual Naval Hospital (http://web.archive.org/web/20051123000128/http://www.vnh.org/FSManual/02/02SustainedAcceleration.html)

[4] Web Archive: Aircraft air quality (http://web.archive.org/web/20061005203309/http://www.house.gov/transportation/aviation/06-05-03/friend.html)

[5] Web Archive: Virtual Naval Hospital, Oxygen Toxity (http://web.archive.org/web/20051122223954/http://www.vnh.org/FSManual/01/10OxygenToxic.html)

[6] Web Archive: Aircraf air quality (http://web.archive.org/web/20061005203309/http://www.house.gov/transportation/aviation/06-05-03/friend.html)

Blindness

Blindness	
Classification and external resources	

A white cane, the international symbol of blindness

ICD-10	H 54.0 [1], H 54.1 [2], H 54.4 [3]
ICD-9	369 [4]
DiseasesDB	28256 [5]

Blindness is the condition of lacking visual perception due to physiological or neurological factors.

Various scales have been developed to describe the extent of vision loss and define blindness.[6] **Total blindness** is the complete lack of form and visual light perception and is clinically recorded as NLP, an abbreviation for "no light perception."[6] *Blindness* is frequently used to describe severe visual impairment with residual vision. Those described as having only light perception have no more sight than the ability to tell light from dark and the general direction of a light source.

In order to determine which people may need special assistance because of their visual disabilities, various governmental jurisdictions have formulated more complex definitions referred to as **legal blindness**.[7] In North America and most of Europe, legal blindness is defined as visual acuity (vision) of 20/200 (6/60) or less in the better eye with best correction possible. This means that a legally blind individual would have to stand 20 feet (6.1 m) from an object to see it—with corrective lenses—with the same degree of clarity as a normally sighted person could from 200 feet (61 m). In many areas, people with average acuity who nonetheless have a visual field of less than 20 degrees (the norm being 180 degrees) are also classified as being legally blind. Approximately ten percent of those deemed legally blind, by any measure, have no vision. The rest have some vision, from light perception alone to relatively good acuity. Low vision is sometimes used to describe visual acuities from 20/70 to 20/200.[8]

By the 10th Revision of the WHO International Statistical Classification of Diseases, Injuries and Causes of Death, *low vision* is defined as visual acuity of less than 20/60 (6/18), but equal to or better than 20/200 (6/60), or corresponding visual field loss to less than 20 degrees, in the better eye with best possible correction. *Blindness* is defined as visual acuity of less than 20/400 (6/120), or corresponding visual field loss to less than 10 degrees, in the better eye with best possible correction.[9] [10]

Blind people with undamaged eyes may still register light non-visually for the purpose of circadian entrainment to the 24-hour light/dark cycle. Light signals for this purpose travel through the retinohypothalamic tract, so a damaged optic nerve beyond where the retinohypothalamic tract exits it is no hindrance.

Classification

In 1934, the American Medical Association adopted the following definition of blindness:

> Central visual acuity of 20/200 or less in the better eye with corrective glasses or central visual acuity of more than 20/200 if there is a visual field defect in which the peripheral field is contracted to such an extent that the widest diameter of the visual field subtends an angular distance no greater than 20 degrees in the better eye.[11]

The United States Congress included this definition as part of the Aid to the Blind program in the Social Security Act passed in 1935.[11] [12] In 1972, the Aid to the Blind program and two others combined under Title XVI of the Social Security Act to form the Supplemental Security Income program[13] which currently states:

> An individual shall be considered to be blind for purposes of this title if he has central visual acuity of 20/200 or less in the better eye with the use of a correcting lens. An eye which is accompanied by a limitation in the fields of vision such that the widest diameter of the visual field subtends an angle no greater than 20 degrees shall be considered for purposes of the first sentence of this subsection as having a central visual acuity of 20/200 or less. An individual shall also be considered to be blind for purposes of this title if he is blind as defined under a State plan approved under title X or XVI as in effect for October 1972 and received aid under such plan (on the basis of blindness) for December 1973, so long as he is continuously blind as so defined.[14]

In the United States, legal blindness due to acuity loss is most often measured by a regular eye doctor with an eye chart.

Legal blindness due to visual field being less than 20 degrees is measured by a visual field test using a number IV target size. If the doctor or facility performing the test is approved by the Social Security Administration, this is the official US determination for legal blindness due to field loss in conditions like retinitis pigmentosa.

Kuwait is one of many nations that share the same criteria for legal blindness.[15]

In the UK, the Certificate of Vision Impairment (CVI) is used to certify patients as severely sight impaired or sight impaired.[16] The accompanying guidance for clinical staff states:

> The National Assistance Act 1948 states that a person can be certified as severely sight impaired if they are "so blind as to be as to be unable to perform any work for which eye sight is essential" (National Assistance Act Section 64(1)). The test is whether a person cannot do any work for which eyesight is essential, not just his or her normal job or one particular job.[17]

In practice, the definition depends on individuals' visual acuity and the extent to which their field of vision is restricted. The Department of Health identifies three groups of patients who may be classified as severely visually impaired.[17]

1. Those below 3/60 Snellen (most people below 3/60 are severely sight impaired),
2. Those better than 3/60 but below 6/60 Snellen (people who have a very contracted field of vision only),
3. Those 6/60 Snellen or above (people in this group who have a contracted field of vision especially if the contraction is in the lower part of the field),

The Department of Health also state that a person is more likely to be classified as severely visually impaired if their eyesight has failed recently or if they are an older individual, both groups being perceived as less able to adapt to their vision loss.[17]

Causes

Serious visual impairment has a variety of causes:

Diseases

According to WHO estimates, the most common causes of blindness around the world in 2002 were:

1. cataracts (47.9%),
2. glaucoma (12.3%),
3. age-related macular degeneration (8.7%),
4. corneal opacity (5.1%), and
5. diabetic retinopathy (4.8%),

6. childhood blindness (3.9%),
7. trachoma (3.6%)
8. onchocerciasis (0.8%).[18]

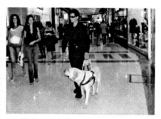

A blind man is led by a guide dog in Brasília, Brazil.

In terms of the worldwide prevalence of blindness, the vastly greater number of people in the developing world and the greater likelihood of their being affected mean that the causes of blindness in those areas are numerically more important. Cataract is responsible for more than 22 million cases of blindness and glaucoma 6 million, while leprosy and onchocerciasis each blind approximately 1 million individuals worldwide. The number of individuals blind from trachoma has dropped dramatically in the past 10 years from 6 million to 1.3 million, putting it in seventh place on the list of causes of blindness worldwide. Xerophthalmia is estimated to affect 5 million children each year; 500,000 develop active corneal involvement, and half of these go blind. Central corneal ulceration is also a significant cause of monocular blindness worldwide, accounting for an estimated 850,000 cases of corneal blindness every year in the Indian subcontinent alone. As a result, corneal scarring from all causes now is the fourth greatest cause of global blindness (Vaughan & Asbury's General Ophthalmology, 17e)

People in developing countries are significantly more likely to experience visual impairment as a consequence of treatable or preventable conditions than are their counterparts in the developed world. While vision impairment is most common in people over age 60 across all regions, children in poorer communities are more likely to be affected by blinding diseases than are their more affluent peers.

The link between poverty and treatable visual impairment is most obvious when conducting regional comparisons of cause. Most adult visual impairment in North America and Western Europe is related to age-related macular degeneration and diabetic retinopathy. While both of these conditions are subject to treatment, neither can be cured.

In developing countries, wherein people have shorter life expectancies, cataracts and water-borne parasites—both of which can be treated effectively—are most often the culprits (see river blindness, for example). Of the estimated 40 million blind people located around the world, 70–80% can have some or all of their sight restored through treatment.

In developed countries where parasitic diseases are less common and cataract surgery is more available, age-related macular degeneration, glaucoma, and diabetic retinopathy are usually the leading causes of blindness.[19]

Childhood blindness can be caused by conditions related to pregnancy, such as congenital rubella syndrome and retinopathy of prematurity.

Abnormalities and injuries

Eye injuries, most often occurring in people under 30, are the leading cause of monocular blindness (vision loss in one eye) throughout the United States. Injuries and cataracts affect the eye itself, while abnormalities such as optic nerve hypoplasia affect the nerve bundle that sends signals from the eye to the back of the brain, which can lead to decreased visual acuity.

People with injuries to the occipital lobe of the brain can, despite having undamaged eyes and optic nerves, still be legally or totally blind.

Genetic defects

People with albinism often have vision loss to the extent that many are legally blind, though few of them actually cannot see. Leber's congenital amaurosis can cause total blindness or severe sight loss from birth or early childhood.

Recent advances in mapping of the human genome have identified other genetic causes of low vision or blindness. One such example is Bardet-Biedl syndrome.

Poisoning

Rarely, blindness is caused by the intake of certain chemicals. A well-known example is methanol, which is only mildly toxic and minimally intoxicating, but when not competing with ethanol for metabolism, methanol breaks down into the substances formaldehyde and formic acid which in turn can cause blindness, an array of other health complications, and death.[20] Methanol is commonly found in methylated spirits, denatured ethyl alcohol, to avoid paying taxes on selling ethanol intended for human consumption. Methylated spirits are sometimes used by alcoholics as a desperate and cheap substitute for regular ethanol alcoholic beverages.

Willful actions

Blinding has been used as an act of vengeance and torture in some instances, to deprive a person of a major sense by which they can navigate or interact within the world, act fully independently, and be aware of events surrounding them. An example from the classical realm is Oedipus, who gouges out his own eyes after realizing that he fulfilled the awful prophecy spoken of him.

In 2003, a Pakistani anti-terrorism court sentenced a man to be blinded after he carried out an acid attack against his fiancee that resulted in her blinding.[21] The same sentence was given in 2009 for the man who blinded Ameneh Bahrami.

Comorbidities

Blindness can occur in combination with such conditions as mental retardation, autism spectrum disorders, cerebral palsy, hearing impairments, and epilepsy.[22] [23] In a study of 228 visually impaired children in metropolitan Atlanta between 1991 and 1993, 154 (68%) had an additional disability besides visual impairment.[22] Blindness in combination with hearing loss is known as deafblindness.

Management

A 2008 study published in the New England Journal of Medicine[24] tested the effect of using gene therapy to help restore the sight of patients with a rare form of inherited blindness, known as Leber Congenital Amaurosis or LCA. Leber Congenital Amaurosis damages the light receptors in the retina and usually begins affecting sight in early childhood, with worsening vision until complete blindness around the age of 30.

The study used a common cold virus to deliver a normal version of the gene called RPE65 directly into the eyes of affected patients. Remarkably all 3 patients aged 19, 22 and 25 responded well to the treatment and reported improved vision following the procedure. Due to the age of the patients and the degenerative nature of LCA the improvement of vision in gene therapy patients is encouraging for researchers. It is hoped that gene therapy may be even more effective in younger LCA patients who have experienced limited vision loss as well as in other blind or partially blind individuals.

Two experimental treatments for retinal problems include a cybernetic replacement and transplant of fetal retinal cells.[25]

Adaptive techniques and aids

Mobility

Many people with serious visual impairments can travel independently, using a wide range of tools and techniques. Orientation and mobility specialists are professionals who are specifically trained to teach people with visual impairments how to travel safely, confidently, and independently in the home and the community. These professionals can also help blind people to practice travelling on specific routes which they may use often, such as the route from one's house to a convenience store. Becoming familiar with an environment or route can make it much easier for a blind person to navigate successfully.

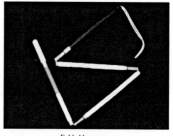
Folded long cane.

Tools such as the white cane with a red tip - the international symbol of blindness - may also be used to improve mobility. A long cane is used to extend the user's range of touch sensation. It is usually swung in a low sweeping motion, across the intended path of travel, to detect obstacles. However, techniques for cane travel can vary depending on the user and/or the situation. Some visually impaired persons do not carry these kinds of canes, opting instead for the shorter, lighter identification (ID) cane. Still others require a support cane. The choice depends on the individual's vision, motivation, and other factors.

A small number of people employ guide dogs to assist in mobility. These dogs are trained to navigate around various obstacles, and to indicate when it becomes necessary to go up or down a step. However, the helpfulness of guide dogs is limited by the inability of dogs to understand complex directions. The human half of the guide dog team does the directing, based upon skills acquired through previous mobility training. In this sense, the handler might be likened to an aircraft's navigator, who must know how to get from one place to another, and the dog to the pilot, who gets them there safely.

Some blind people use GPS for the visually impaired as a mobility aid. Such software can assist blind people with orientation and navigation, but it is not a replacement for traditional mobility tools such as white canes and guide dogs.

Technology to allow blind people to drive motor vehicles is currently being developed.[26]

Government actions are sometimes taken to make public places more accessible to blind people. Public transportation is freely available to the blind in many cities. Tactile paving and audible traffic signals can make it easier and safer for visually impaired pedestrians to cross streets. In addition to making rules about who can and cannot use a cane, some governments mandate the right-of-way be given to users of white canes or guide dogs.

Reading and magnification

Most visually impaired people who are not totally blind read print, either of a regular size or enlarged by magnification devices. Many also read large-print, which is easier for them to read without such devices. A variety of magnifying glasses, some handheld, and some on desktops, can make reading easier for them.

Others read Braille (or the infrequently used Moon type), or rely on talking books and readers or reading machines, which convert printed text to speech or Braille. They use computers with special hardware such as scanners and refreshable Braille displays as well as software written specifically for the blind, such as optical character recognition applications and screen readers.

Some people access these materials through agencies for the blind, such as the National Library Service for the Blind and Physically Handicapped in the United States, the National Library for the Blind or the RNIB in the United Kingdom.

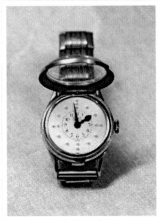

Braille watch

Closed-circuit televisions, equipment that enlarges and contrasts textual items, are a more high-tech alternative to traditional magnification devices.

There are also over 100 radio reading services throughout the world that provide people with vision impairments with readings from periodicals over the radio. The International Association of Audio Information Services provides links to all of these organizations.

Computers

Access technology such as screen readers, screen magnifiers and refreshable Braille displays enable the blind to use mainstream computer applications and mobile phones. The availability of assistive technology is increasing, accompanied by concerted efforts to ensure the accessibility of information technology to all potential users, including the blind. Later versions of Microsoft Windows include an Accessibility Wizard & Magnifier for those with partial vision, and Microsoft Narrator, a simple screen reader. Linux distributions (as live CDs) for the blind include Oralux and Adriane Knoppix, the latter developed in part by Adriane Knopper who has a visual impairment. Mac OS also comes with a built-in screen reader, called VoiceOver.

The movement towards greater web accessibility is opening a far wider number of websites to adaptive technology, making the web a more inviting place for visually impaired surfers.

Experimental approaches in sensory substitution are beginning to provide access to arbitrary live views from a camera.

Other aids and techniques

Blind people may use talking equipment such as thermometers, watches, clocks, scales, calculators, and compasses. They may also enlarge or mark dials on devices such as ovens and thermostats to make them usable. Other techniques used by blind people to assist them in daily activities include:

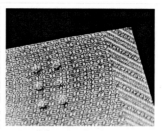

A tactile feature on a Canadian banknote.

- Adaptations of coins and banknotes so that the value can be determined by touch. For example:

  - In some currencies, such as the euro, the pound sterling and the Indian rupee, the size of a note increases with its value.
  - On US coins, pennies and dimes, and nickels and quarters are similar in size. The larger denominations (dimes and quarters) have ridges along the sides (historically used to prevent the "shaving" of precious metals from the coins), which can now be used for identification.
  - Some currencies' banknotes have a tactile feature to indicate denomination. For example, the Canadian currency tactile feature is a system of raised dots in one corner, based on Braille cells but not standard Braille.[27]
    - It is also possible to fold notes in different ways to assist recognition.
- Labeling and tagging clothing and other personal items
- Placing different types of food at different positions on a dinner plate
- Marking controls of household appliances

Most people, once they have been visually impaired for long enough, devise their own adaptive strategies in all areas of personal and professional management.

Epidemiology

The WHO estimates that in 2002 there were 161 million visually impaired people in the world (about 2.6% of the total population). Of this number 124 million (about 2%) had low vision and 37 million (about 0.6%) were blind.[28] In order of frequency the leading causes were cataract, uncorrected refractive errors (near sighted, far sighted, or an astigmatism), glaucoma, and age-related macular degeneration.[29] In 1987, it was estimated that 598,000 people in the United States met the legal definition of blindness.[30] Of this number, 58% were over the age of 65.[30] In 1994-1995, 1.3 million Americans reported legal blindness.[31]

Society and culture

Metaphorical uses

The word "blind" (adjective and verb) is often used to signify a lack of knowledge of something. For example, a blind date is a date in which the people involved have not previously met; a blind experiment is one in which information is kept from either the experimenter or the participant in order to mitigate the placebo effect or observer bias. The expression "blind leading the blind" refers to incapable people leading other incapable people. Being blind to something means not understanding or being aware of it. A "blind spot" is an area where someone cannot see, e.g. where a car driver cannot see because parts of his car's bodywork are in the way.

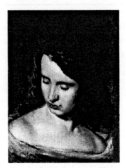

Portrait of a *Blind woman* by Diego Velázquez.

Sports

Blind and partially sighted people participate in sports such as swimming, snow skiing and athletics. Some sports have been invented or adapted for the blind such as goalball, association football, cricket, and golf.[32] The worldwide authority on sports for the blind is the International Blind Sports Federation.[33] People with vision impairments have participated in the Paralympic Games since the 1976 summer Paralympics in Toronto.[34]

In other animals

Statements that certain species of mammals are "born blind" refers to them being born with their eyes closed and their eyelids fused together; the eyes open later. One example is the rabbit. In humans the eyelids are fused for a while before birth, but open again before the normal birth time, but very premature babies are sometimes born with their eyes fused shut, and opening later. Other animals such as the blind mole rat are truly blind and rely on other senses.

The theme of blind animals has been a powerful one in literature. Peter Schaffer's Tony-Award winning play, Equus, tells the story of a boy who blinds six horses. Theodore Taylor's classic young adult novel, *The Trouble With Tuck*, is about a teenage girl, Helen, who trains her blind dog to follow and trust a seeing-eye dog. Jacob Appel's prize-winning story, "Rods and Cones," describes the disruption that a blind rabbit causes in a married couple's life. In non-fiction, a recent classic is Linda Kay Hardie's essay, "Lessons Learned from a Blind Cat," in *Cat Women: Female Writers on their Feline Friends*.

References

[1] http://apps.who.int/classifications/apps/icd/icd10online/?gh53.htm+h540

[2] http://apps.who.int/classifications/apps/icd/icd10online/?gh53.htm+h541

[3] http://apps.who.int/classifications/apps/icd/icd10online/?gh53.htm+h544

[4] http://www.icd9data.com/getICD9Code.ashx?icd9=369

[5] http://www.diseasesdatabase.com/ddb28256.htm

[6] International Council of Ophthalmology. "International Standards: Visual Standards — Aspects and Ranges of Vision Loss with Emphasis on Population Surveys." (http://www.icoph.org/pdf/visualstandardsreport.pdf) April 2002.

[7] Belote, Larry. "Low Vision Education and Training: Defining the Boundaries of Low Vision Patients." (http://www.larrybelote.com/Files/Low Vision Education and Training/Extending the Boundaries of Service.DOC) *A Personal Guide to the VA Visual Impairment Services Program.* Retrieved March 31, 2006.

[8] Living with Low Vision - American Foundation for the Blind (http://www.afb.org/Section.asp?SectionID=26&TopicID=144)

[9] http://www3.who.int/icd/currentversion/fr-icd.htm

[10] WHO | Magnitude and causes of visual impairment (http://www.who.int/mediacentre/factsheets/fs282/en/)

[11] Koestler, F. A., (1976). *The unseen minority: a social history of blindness in the United States.* New York: David McKay.

[12] Corn, AL; Spungin, SJ. "Free and Appropriate Public Education and the Personnel Crisis for Students with Visual Impairments and Blindness." (http://www.coe.ufl.edu/copsse/docs/IB-10/1/IB-10.pdf) Center on Personnel Studies in Special Education. April 2003.

[13] http://www.ssa.gov/history/pdf/80chap12.pdf

[14] Social Security Act. "Sec. 1614. Meaning of terms." (http://www.ssa.gov/OP_Home/ssact/title16b/1614.htm) Retrieved February 17, 2006.

[15] Al-Merjan, JI; Pandova, MG; Al-Ghanim, M; Al-Wayel, A; Al-Mutairi, S (2005). "Registered blindness and low vision in Kuwait". *Ophthalmic epidemiology* **12** (4): 251–7. doi:10.1080/09286580591005813. PMID 16033746.

[16] "Identification and notification of sight loss" (http://www.dh.gov.uk/en/Healthcare/Primarycare/Optical/DH_4074843) Retrieved April 26, 2010.

[17] "Certificate of Vision Impairment: Explanatory Notes for Consultant Ophthalmologists and Hospital Eye Clinic Staff" (http://www.dh.gov.uk/prod_consum_dh/groups/dh_digitalassets/documents/digitalasset/dh_078294.pdf) retrieved April 26, 2010.

[18] "Causes of blindness and visual impairment" (http://www.who.int/blindness/causes/en/). World Health Organization. . Retrieved 19 February 2009.

[19] Bunce, C; Wormald, R (2006). "Leading causes of certification for blindness and partial sight in England & Wales" (http://www.pubmedcentral.nih.gov/articlerender.fcgi?tool=pmcentrez&artid=1420283). *BMC public health* **6**: 58. doi:10.1186/1471-2458-6-58. PMID 16524463. PMC 1420283.

[20] "Methanol" (http://web.archive.org/web/20070220004549/http://www.safety-council.org/info/OSH/methanol.htm) (Web). *Symptoms of Methanol Poisoning.* Canada Safety Council. 2005. Archived from the original (http://www.safety-council.org/info/OSH/methanol.htm) on February 20, 2007. . Retrieved March 27, 2007.

[21] "Eye-for-eye in Pakistan acid case" (http://news.bbc.co.uk/2/hi/south_asia/3313207.stm). BBC News. 12 December 2003. . Retrieved 2008-06-30.

[22] "Causes of Blindness" (http://www.lighthouse.org/about-low-vision-blindness/causes-of-blindness/). Lighthouse International. . Retrieved 27 May 2010.

[23] "Autism and Blindness" (http://www.ncecbvi.org/autism.htm). Nerbraska Center for the Education of Children who are Blind or Visually Impaired. . Retrieved 27 May 2010.

[24] Bainbridge JW, Smith AJ, Barker SS, *et al.* (May 2008). "Effect of gene therapy on visual function in Leber's congenital amaurosis" (http://content.nejm.org/cgi/content/abstract/NEJMoa0802268). *N. Engl. J. Med.* **358** (21): 2231–9. doi:10.1056/NEJMoa0802268. PMID 18441371. .

[25] Bionic Eye Opens New World Of Sight For Blind (http://www.npr.org/templates/story/story.php?storyId=113968653) by Jon Hamilton. All Things Considered, National Public Radio. 20 October 2009.

[26] ["Blind driver to debut new technologies at Daytona" (http://news.yahoo.com/s/ap/20110128/ap_on_re_us/us_blind_driver). Associated Press. 28 January 2011. [http://news.yahoo.com/s/ap/20110128/ap_on_re_us/us_blind_driver. Retrieved 29 January 2011.

[27] Accessibility features - Bank Notes - Bank of Canada (http://www.bankofcanada.ca/en/banknotes/accessibility.html)

[28] "World Health Organization" (http://www.who.int/en/) (Web). World Health Organization. 2006. . Retrieved December 16, 2006.

[29] "WHO | Visual impairment and blindness" (http://www.who.int/mediacentre/factsheets/fs282/en/index.html). .

[30] Kirchner, C., Stephen, G. & Chandu, F. (1987). "Estimated 1987 prevalence of non-institutionalized 'severe visual impairment' by age base on 1977 estimated rates: U. S.", 1987. *AER Yearbook.*

[31] American Foundation for the Blind. "Statistics and Sources for Professionals." (http://www.afb.org/Section.asp?SectionID=15&DocumentID=1367#prev) Retrieved April 1, 2006.

[32] "Blind Sports Victoria" (http://www.blindsports.org.au/). . Retrieved 2008-03-04.

[33] "IBSA General Assembly Elects New Leadership" (http://www.paralympic.org/paralympian/20014/2001430.htm). *The Paralympian.* International Paralympic Committee. April 2001. . Retrieved 2008-03-04.

[34] "The history of people with disabilities in Australia - 100 years" (http://www.dsa.org.au/life_site/text/sport/index.html). Disability Services Australia. . Retrieved 2008-03-04.

External links

• Blindness Resource Center (http://www.nyise.org/blind.htm) from The New York Institute for Special Education

bjn:Picak

Dystrophy

Dystrophy is any condition of abnormal development, often denoting the degeneration of muscles.

Types

- Muscular dystrophy
- Duchenne muscular dystrophy
- Becker's muscular dystrophy
- Reflex neurovascular dystrophy
- Retinal dystrophy
- Conal dystrophy
- Myotonic dystrophy
- Corneal dystrophies

Photoreceptor cell

Neuron: Photoreceptor Cell
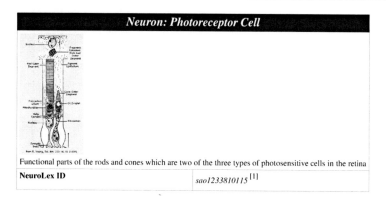
Functional parts of the rods and cones which are two of the three types of photosensitive cells in the retina
NeuroLex ID	$sao1233810115$ [1]

A **photoreceptor**, or **photoreceptor cell**, is a specialized type of neuron (nerve cell) found in the eye's retina that is capable of phototransduction. The great biological importance of photoreceptors is that as cells they convert light (electromagnetic radiation) into the beginning of a chain of biological processes. More specifically, the photoreceptor absorbs photons from the field of view, and through a specific and complex biochemical pathway, signals this information through a change in its membrane potential.

For hundreds of years, photoreceptors in vertebrates were thought to be of only two main classes. The two classic photoreceptors are rods and cones, each contributing information used by the visual system to form a representation of the visual world, sight. The rods are slightly narrower than the cones but are similarly formed.[2] A third class of photoreceptors was discovered during the 1990s:[3] the photosensitive ganglion cells. These cells, found in the inner retina, have dendrites and long axons projecting to several areas of the brain.

There are major functional differences between the rods and cones. Cones are adapted to detect colors, and function well in bright light; rods are more sensitive, but do not detect color well, being adapted for low light. In humans there are three different types of cone — responding respectively to short (blue), medium (green) and long (yellow-red) light. The human retina contains about 120 million rod cells and 6 million cone cells. The number and ratio of rods to cones varies among species, dependent on whether an animal is primarily diurnal or nocturnal. Certain owls have a tremendous number of rods in their retinas — the eyes of the tawny owl are approximately 100 times more sensitive at night than those of humans.[4] There are about 1.3 million ganglion cells in the human visual system; 1 to 2% of them are photosensitive.

Described here are vertebrate photoreceptors. Invertebrate photoreceptors in organisms such as insects and molluscs are different in both their morphological organization and their underlying biochemical pathways.

Histology

Rod and cone photoreceptors have the same complex structural formation. Closest to the visual field (and farthest from the brain) is the axon terminal, which releases a neurotransmitter called glutamate to bipolar cells. Farther back is the cell body, which contains the cell's organelles. Farther back still is the inner segment, a specialized part of the cell full of mitochondria. The chief function of the inner segment is to provide ATP (energy) for the sodium-potassium pump. Finally, closest to the brain (and farthest from the field of view) is the outer segment, the part of the photoreceptor that absorbs light. Outer segments are actually modified cilia that contain disks filled with opsin, the molecule that absorbs photons, as well as voltage-gated sodium channels.

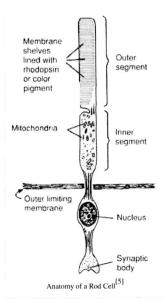

Anatomy of a Rod Cell[5]

The membranous photoreceptor protein *opsin* contains a pigment molecule called *retinal*. In rod cells, these together are called rhodopsin. In cone cells there are different types of opsins that combine with retinal to form pigments called photopsins. Three different classes of photopsins in the cones react to different ranges of light frequency, a differentiation which eventually allows the visual system to distinguish color. The function of the photoreceptor cell is to convert the light energy of the photon into a form of energy communicable to the nervous system and readily usable to the organism: this conversion is called signal transduction.

The opsin found in the photosensitive ganglion cells of the retina that are involved in various reflexive responses of the brain and body to the presence of (day)light, such as the regulation of circadian rhythms, pupillary reflex and other non-visual responses to light, is called melanopsin. Atypical in vertebrates, melanopsin functionally resembles invertebrate opsins. In structure, it is an opsin, a retinylidene protein variety of G-protein-coupled receptor.

When light activates the melanopsin signaling system, the melanopsin-containing ganglion cells discharge nerve impulses which are conducted through their axons to specific brain targets. These targets include the olivary pretectal nucleus (a center responsible for controlling the pupil of the eye), the LGN, and, through the retinohypothalamic tract (RHT), the suprachiasmatic nucleus of the hypothalamus (the master pacemaker of circadian rhythms). Melanopsin-containing ganglion cells are thought to influence these targets by releasing from their axon terminals the neurotransmitters glutamate and pituitary adenylate cyclase activating polypeptide (PACAP).

Humans

The human visual system uses millions of photoreceptors. All photoreceptors in humans are found in the retina at the back of each eye; the ocular photoreceptors and the melanopsin-containing photosensitive ganglion cells are the only neurons capable of phototransduction in humans. The rods and cones are in the outer nuclear layer while the bipolar and ganglion cells that transmit information from photoreceptors to the brain are in front of them. This inverted arrangement significantly reduces acuity, as light must travel through the axons and cell bodies of other neurons before reaching the photoreceptors. The retina contains two specializations to deal with this issue. First, a region at the center of the retina, called the fovea, containing only photoreceptors, is used for high visual acuity. Second, each retina contains a blind spot, an area where axons from the ganglion cells can go back through the retina to the brain.

For hundreds of years. humans were thought to have only the two types of retinal photoreceptors involved in image-forming vision: rods and cones. Both transduce light into a change in membrane potential through the same signal transduction pathway (see below). However, they differ in the nature of the opsin they contain, and their functions. Rods are used primarily to see at low levels of light, while cones are used to determine color, depth, and intensity. Furthermore, there are three types of cones, which differ in the spectrum of wavelengths of photons over which they absorb (see graph). Because cones respond to both the

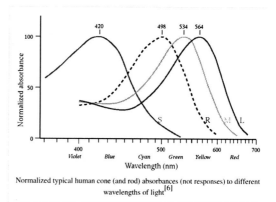

Normalized typical human cone (and rod) absorbances (not responses) to different wavelengths of light[6]

wavelength and intensity of light, a single cone cannot tell color; instead, color vision requires interactions of more than one type of cone (see below), primarily by comparing responses across different cone types.

Phototransduction

Phototransduction is the complex process whereby the energy of a photon is used to change the inherent membrane potential of the photoreceptor. This change thereby signals to the nervous system that light is in the visual field.

Activation of rods and cones is actually hyperpolarization; when they are not being stimulated, they depolarize and release glutamate continuously. In the dark, cells have a relatively high concentration of cyclic guanosine 3'-5' monophosphate (cGMP), which opens ion channels (largely sodium channels, though calcium can enter through these channels as well). The positive charges of the ions that enter the cell down its electrochemical gradient change the cell's membrane potential, cause depolarization, and lead to the release of the neurotransmitter glutamate. Glutamate can depolarize some neurons and hyperpolarize others.

When light hits a photoreceptive pigment within the photoreceptor cell, the pigment changes shape. The pigment, called iodopsin or rhodopsin, consists of large proteins called opsin (situated in the plasma membrane), attached to a covalently-bound prosthetic group: an organic molecule called retinal (a derivative of vitamin A). The retinal exists in the 11-cis-retinal form when in the dark, and stimulation by light causes its structure to change to all-trans-retinal. This structural change causes it to activate a regulatory protein called transducin, which leads to the activation of cGMP phosphodiesterase, which breaks cGMP down into 5'-GMP. Reduction in cGMP allows the ion channels to close, preventing the influx of positive ions, hyperpolarizing the cell, and stopping the release of neurotransmitters.[7] The entire process by which light initiates a sensory response is called visual phototransduction.

Dark current

Unstimulated (in the dark), cyclic-nucleotide gated channels in the outer segment are open because cyclic GMP (cGMP) is bound to them. Hence, positively charged ions (namely sodium ions) enter the photoreceptor, depolarizing it to about −40 mV (resting potential in other nerve cells is usually −65 mV). This depolarizing current is often known as dark current.

Signal transduction pathway

The signal transduction pathway is the mechanism by which the energy of a photon signals a mechanism in the cell that leads to its electrical polarization. This polarization ultimately leads to either the transmittance or inhibition of a neural signal that will be fed to the brain via the optic nerve. The steps, or signal transduction pathway, in the vertebrate eye's rod and cone photoreceptors are then:

1. The rhodopsin or iodopsin in the outer segment absorbs a photon, changing the configuration of a retinal Schiff base cofactor inside the protein from the cis-form to the trans-form, causing the retinal to change shape.
2. This results in a series of unstable intermediates, the last of which binds stronger to the G protein in the membrane and activates transducin, a protein inside the cell. This is the first amplification step – each photoactivated rhodopsin triggers activation of about 100 transducins. (The shape change in the opsin activates a G protein called transducin.)
3. Each transducin then activates the enzyme cGMP-specific phosphodiesterase (PDE).
4. PDE then catalyzes the hydrolysis of cGMP. This is the second amplification step, where a single PDE hydrolyses about 1000 cGMP molecules. (The enzyme hydrolyzes the second messenger cGMP to GMP)
5. With the intracellular concentration of cGMP reduced, the net result is closing of cyclic nucleotide-gated ion channels in the photoreceptor membrane because cGMP was keeping the channels open. (Because cGMP acts to keep Na^+ ion channels open, the conversion of cGMP to GMP closes the channels.)
6. As a result, sodium ions can no longer enter the cell, and the photoreceptor hyperpolarizes (its charge inside the membrane becomes more negative). (The closing of Na^+ channels hyperpolarizes the cell.)
7. This change in the cell's membrane potential causes voltage-gated calcium channels to close. This leads to a decrease in the influx of calcium ions into the cell and thus the intracellular calcium ion concentration falls.
8. The lack of calcium means that less glutamate is released to the bipolar cell than before (see below). (The decreased calcium level slows the release of the neurotransmitter glutamate, which can either excite or inhibit the postsynaptic bipolar cells.)
9. Reduction in the release of glutamate means one population of bipolar cells will be depolarized and a separate population of bipolar cells will be hyperpolarized, depending on the nature of receptors (ionotropic or metabotropic) in the postsynaptic terminal (see receptive field).

Thus, a rod or cone photoreceptor actually releases less neurotransmitter when stimulated by light.

ATP provided by the inner segment powers the sodium-potassium pump. This pump is necessary to reset the initial state of the outer segment by taking the sodium ions that are entering the cell and pumping them back out.

Although photoreceptors are neurons, they do not conduct action potentials with the exception of the photosensitive ganglion cell -which are mainly involved in the regulation of circadian rhythms, melatonin, and control of pupil dilation.

Advantages

Phototransduction in rods and cones is unique in that the stimulus (in this case, light) actually reduces the cell's response or firing rate, which is unusual for a sensory system where the stimulus usually increases the cell's response or firing rate. However, this system offers several key advantages.

First, the classic (rod or cone) photoreceptor is depolarized in the dark, which means many sodium ions are flowing into the cell. Thus, the random opening or closing of sodium channels will not affect the membrane potential of the cell; only the closing of a large number of channels, through absorption of a photon, will affect it and signal that light is in the visual field. Hence, the system is noiseless.

Second, there is a lot of amplification in two stages of classic phototransduction: one pigment will activate many molecules of transducin, and one PDE will cleave many cGMPs. This amplification means that even the absorption of one photon will affect membrane potential and signal to the brain that light is in the visual field. This is the main feature which differentiates rod photoreceptors from cone photoreceptors. Rods are extremely sensitive and have the capacity of registering a single photon of light unlike cones. On the other hand, cones are known to have very fast kinetics in terms of rate of amplification of phototransduction unlike rods.

Difference between rods and cones

Comparison of human rod and cone cells, from Eric Kandel et al. in *Principles of Neural Science*.[7]

Rods	Cones
Used for scotopic vision	Used for photopic vision
Very light sensitive; sensitive to scattered light	Not very light sensitive; sensitive to only direct light
Loss causes night blindness	Loss causes legal blindness
Low visual acuity	High visual acuity; better spatial resolution
Not present in fovea	Concentrated in fovea
Slow response to light, stimuli added over time	Fast response to light, can perceive more rapid changes in stimuli
Have more pigment than cones, so can detect lower light levels	Have less pigment than rods, require more light to detect images
Stacks of membrane-enclosed disks are unattached to cell membrane directly	Disks are attached to outer membrane
20 times more rods than cones in the retina	
One type of photosensitive pigment	Three types of photosensitive pigment in humans
Confer achromatic vision	Confer color vision

Function

Photoreceptors do not signal color; they only signal the presence of light in the visual field.

A given photoreceptor responds to both the wavelength and intensity of a light source. For example, red light at a certain intensity can produce the same exact response in a photoreceptor as green light of a different intensity. Therefore, the response of a single photoreceptor is ambiguous when it comes to color.

To determine color, the visual system compares responses across a population of photoreceptors (specifically, the three different cones with differing absorption spectra). To determine intensity, the visual system computes how many photoreceptors are responding. This is the mechanism that allows trichromatic color vision in humans and some other animals.

Signaling

The rod and cone photoreceptors signal their absorption of photons through a release of the neurotransmitter glutamate to bipolar cells at its axon terminal. Since the photoreceptor is depolarized in the dark, a high amount of glutamate is being released to bipolar cells in the dark. Absorption of a photon will hyperpolarize the photoreceptor and therefore result in the release of *less* glutamate at the presynaptic terminal to the bipolar cell.

Every rod or cone photoreceptor releases the same neurotransmitter, glutamate. However, the effect of glutamate differs in the bipolar cells, depending upon the type of receptor imbedded in that cell's membrane. When glutamate binds to an ionotropic receptor, the bipolar cell will depolarize (and therefore will hyperpolarize with light as less glutamate is released). On the other hand, binding of glutamate to a metabotropic receptor results in a hyperpolarization, so this bipolar cell will depolarize to light as less glutamate is released.

In essence, this property allows for one population of bipolar cells that gets excited by light and another population that gets inhibited by it, even though all photoreceptors show the same response to light. This complexity becomes both important and necessary for detecting color, contrast, edges, etc.

Further complexity arises from the various interconnections among bipolar cells, horizontal cells, and amacrine cells in the retina. The final result is differing populations of ganglion cells in the retina, a sub-population of which is also intrinsically photosensitive, using the photopigment melanopsin.

Ganglion cell (non-rod non-cone) photoreceptors

A non-rod non-cone photoreceptor in the eyes of mice, which was shown to mediate circadian rhythms, was discovered in 1991 by Foster *et al.*[3] These neuronal cells, called intrinsically photosensitive retinal ganglion cells (ipRGC), are a small subset (~1–3%) of the retinal ganglion cells located in the inner retina, that is, in front[8] of the rods and cones located in the outer retina. These light sensitive neurons contain a photopigment, melanopsin,[9] [10] [11] [12] [13] which has an absorption peak of the light at a different wavelength (~480 nm[14]) than rods and cones. Beside circadian / behavioral functions, ipRGCs have a role in initiating the pupillary light reflex.[15]

Dennis Dacey with colleagues showed in a species of Old World monkey that giant ganglion cells expressing melanopsin projected to the lateral geniculate nucleus (LGN).[16] Previously only projections to the midbrain (pre-tectal nucleus) and hypothalamus (suprachiasmatic nucleus) had been shown. However a visual role for the receptor was still unsuspected and unproven.

In 2007, Farhan H. Zaidi and colleagues published pioneering work using rodless coneless humans. *Current Biology* subsequently announced in their 2008 editorial, commentary and despatches to scientists and ophthalmologists, that the non-rod non-cone photoreceptor had been conclusively discovered in humans using landmark experiments on rodless coneless humans by Zaidi and colleagues[13] [17] [18] [19] As had been found in other mammals, the identity of the non-rod non-cone photoreceptor in humans was found to be a ganglion cell in the inner retina. The workers had tracked down patients with rare diseases wiping out classic rod and cone photoreceptor function but preserving ganglion cell function.[17] [18] [19] Despite having no rods or cones the patients continued to exhibit circadian photoentrainment, circadian behavioural patterns, melanopsin suppression, and pupil reactions, with peak spectral sensitivities to environmental and experimental light matching that for the melanopsin photopigment. Their brains could also associate vision with light of this frequency.

In humans the retinal ganglion cell photoreceptor contributes to conscious sight as well as to non-image-forming functions like circadian rhythms, behaviour and pupil reactions.[20] Since these cells respond mostly to blue light, it has been suggested that they have a role in mesopic vision. Zaidi and colleagues' work with rodless coneless human subjects hence also opened the door into image-forming (visual) roles for the ganglion cell photoreceptor. It was discovered that there are parallel pathways for vision – one classic rod and cone-based arising from the outer retina, the other a rudimentary visual brightness detector arising from the inner retina and which seems to be activated by light before the other.[20] Classic photoreceptors also feed into the novel photoreceptor system, and colour constancy may be an important role as suggested by Foster. The receptor could be instrumental in understanding many diseases including major causes of blindness worldwide like glaucoma, a disease which affects ganglion cells, and the study of the receptor offered potential as a new avenue to explore in trying to find treatments for blindness. It is in these discoveries of the novel photoreceptor in humans and in the receptors role in vision, rather than its non-image-forming functions, where the receptor may have the greatest impact on society as a whole, though the impact of disturbed circadian rhythms is another area of relevance to clinical medicine.

Most work suggests that the peak spectral sensitivity of the receptor is between 460 and 482 nm. Steven Lockley et al. in 2003 showed that 460 nm wavelengths of light suppress melatonin twice as much as longer 555 nm light. However, in more recent work by Farhan Zaidi et al., using rodless coneless humans, it was found that what consciously led to light perception was a very intense 481 nm stimulus; this means that the receptor in visual terms enables some rudimentary vision maximally for blue light.[20]

Sports

Since rods are much slower to respond to light stimulation than cones, sporting events such as baseball become gradually harder as daylight subsides.[21]

See also

- Visual phototransduction
- G protein-coupled receptor
- Sensory system
- Photosensitive
- Photosensitive ganglion cell
- Horizontal cell
- Bipolar cell
- Amacrine cell

References

[1] http://www.neurolex.org/wiki/sao1233810115
[2] "eye, human." Encyclopædia Britannica. Encyclopaedia Britannica Ultimate Reference Suite. Chicago: Encyclopædia Britannica, 2010.
[3] Foster, R.G.; Provencio, I.; Hudson, D.; Fiske, S.; Grip, W.; Menaker, M. (1991). "Circadian photoreception in the retinally degenerate mouse (rd/rd)". *Journal of Comparative Physiology A* **169**. doi:10.1007/BF00198171.
[4] "Owl Eyesight" (http://www.owls.org/Information/eyesight.htm) at owls.org
[5] Human Physiology and Mechanisms of Disease by Arthur C. Guyton (1992) ISBN 0721632998 p. 373
[6] Bowmaker J.K. and Dartnall H.J.A. (1980). "Visual pigments of rods and cones in a human retina" (http://www.pubmedcentral.nih.gov/articlerender.fcgi?tool=pmcentrez&artid=1279132). *J. Physiol.* **298**: 501–511. PMID 7359434. PMC 1279132.
[7] Kandel, E. R.; Schwartz, J.H.; Jessell, T.M. (2000). *Principles of Neural Science* (4th ed.). New York: McGraw-Hill. pp. 507–513. ISBN 0-8385-7701-6.
[8] See retina for information on the retinal layer structure.
[9] Provencio, I. et al. (2000-01-15). "A human opsin in the inner retina". *The Journal of Neuroscience* **20** (2): 600–605. PMID 10632589.
[10] Hattar, S.; Liao, HW; Takao, M; Berson, DM; Yau, KW (2002). "Melanopsin-Containing Retinal Ganglion Cells: Architecture, Projections, and Intrinsic Photosensitivity" (http://www.pubmedcentral.nih.gov/articlerender.fcgi?tool=pmcentrez&artid=2885915). *Science* **295** (5557): 1065. doi:10.1126/science.1069609. PMID 11834834. PMC 2885915.
[11] Melyan, Z.; Tarttelin, E. E.; Bellingham, J.; Lucas, R. J.; Hankins, M. W. (2005). "Addition of human melanopsin renders mammalian cells photoresponsive". *Nature* **433**: 741. doi:10.1038/nature03344.
[12] Qiu, Xudong; Kumbalasiri, Tida; Carlson, Stephanie M.; Wong, Kwoon Y.; Krishna, Vanitha; Provencio, Ignacio; Berson, David M. (2005). "Induction of photosensitivity by heterologous expression of melanopsin". *Nature* **433** (7027): 745. doi:10.1038/nature03345. PMID 15674243.
[13] Vangelder, R (2008). "Non-Visual Photoreception: Sensing Light without Sight". *Current Biology* **18** (1): R38. doi:10.1016/j.cub.2007.11.027. PMID 18177714.

[14] Berson, David M. (2007). "Phototransduction in ganglion-cell photoreceptors". *Pflügers Archiv - European Journal of Physiology* **454**: 849. doi:10.1007/s00424-007-0242-2.

[15] Lucas, Robert J.; Douglas, Ronald H.; Foster, Russell G. (2001). "Characterization of an ocular photopigment capable of driving pupillary constriction in mice.". *Nature Neuroscience* **4** (6): 621. doi:10.1038/88443. PMID 11369943.

[16] Dacey, Dennis M.; Liao, Hsi-Wen; Peterson, Beth B.; Robinson, Farrel R.; Smith, Vivianne C.; Pokorny, Joel; Yau, King-Wai; Gamlin, Paul D. (2005). "Melanopsin-expressing ganglion cells in primate retina signal colour and irradiance and project to the LGN". *Nature* **433** (7027): 749. doi:10.1038/nature03387. PMID 15716953.

[17] Genova, Cathleen, Blind humans lacking rods and cones retain normal responses to nonvisual effects of light (http://www.eurekalert.org/pub_releases/2007-12/cp-bhl121307.php). Cell Press, December 13, 2007.

[18] Coghlan A. Blind people 'see' sunrise and sunset (http://www.newscientist.com/article/mg19626354.100-blind-people-see-sunrise-and-sunset.html). New Scientist, 26 December 2007, issue 2635.

[19] Medical News Today. Normal Responses To Non-visual Effects Of Light Retained By Blind Humans Lacking Rods And Cones (http://www.medicalnewstoday.com/articles/91836.php). 14 December 2007.

[20] Zaidi FH et al. (2007). "Short-wavelength light sensitivity of circadian, pupillary, and visual awareness in humans lacking an outer retina." (http://www.pubmedcentral.nih.gov/articlerender.fcgi?tool=pmcentrez&artid=2151130). *Current biology : CB* **17** (24): 2122–8. doi:10.1016/j.cub.2007.11.034. PMID 18082405. PMC 2151130.

[21] "Webvision: Photoreceptors" (http://webvision.med.utah.edu/photo2.html). Webvision.med.utah.edu. . Retrieved 2010-12-12.

Bibliography

- Campbell, Neil A., and Reece, Jane B. (2002). *Biology*. San Francisco: Benjamin Cummings. pp. 1064–1067. ISBN 0-8053-6624-5.
- Freeman, Scott (2002). *Biological Science (2nd Edition)*. Englewood Cliffs, N.J: Prentice Hall. pp. 835–837. ISBN 0-13-140941-7.

External links

- NIF Search – Photoreceptor Cell (http://www.neuinfo.org/nif/nifgwt.html?query="Photoreceptor Cell") via the Neuroscience Information Framework

Retinal pigment epithelium

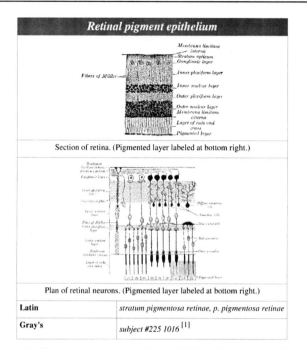

Retinal pigment epithelium	
Section of retina. (Pigmented layer labeled at bottom right.)	
Plan of retinal neurons. (Pigmented layer labeled at bottom right.)	
Latin	*stratum pigmentosa retinae, p. pigmentosa retinae*
Gray's	*subject #225 1016* [1]

The **pigmented layer of retina** or **retinal pigment epithelium** (**RPE**) is the pigmented cell layer just outside the neurosensory retina that nourishes retinal visual cells, and is firmly attached to the underlying choroid and overlying retinal visual cells.[2] [3]

History

The RPE was known in the 18th and 19th centuries as the **pigmentum nigrum,** referring to the observation that the RPE is dark (black in many animals, brown in humans); and as the **tapetum nigrum,** referring to the observation that in animals with a tapetum lucidum, in the region of the tapetum lucidum the RPE is not pigmented.[4]

Anatomy

The RPE is composed of a single layer of hexagonal cells that are densely packed with pigment granules.[2]

At the ora serrata, the RPE continues as a membrane passing over the ciliary body and continuing as the back surface of the iris. This generates the fibers of the dilator. Directly beneath this epithelium is

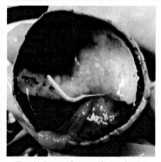

Choroid dissected from a calf's eye, showing black RPE and iridescent blue tapetum lucidum

the neuroepithelium (i.e., rods and cones)passes jointly with the RPE. Both, combined, are understood to be the ciliary epithelium of the embryo. The front end continuaton of the retina is the posterior iris epithelium, which takes on pigment when it enters the iris[5]

When viewed from the outer surface, these cells are smooth and hexagonal in shape. When seen in section, each cell consists of an outer non-pigmented part containing a large oval nucleus and an inner pigmented portion which extends as a series of straight thread-like processes between the rods, this being especially the case when the eye is exposed to light.

Function

The retinal pigment epithelium is involved in the phagocytosis of the outer segment of photoreceptor cells and it is also involved in the vitamin A cycle where it isomerizes all trans retinol to 11-cis retinal.

The retinal pigment epithelium also serves as the limiting transport factor that maintains the retinal environment by supplying small molecules such as amino acid, ascorbic acid and D-glucose while remaining a tight barrier to choroidal blood borne substances. Homeostasis of the ionic environment is maintained by a delicate transport exchange system.

Pathology

In the eyes of albinos, the cells of this layer contain no pigment. Dysfunction of the RPE is found in Age-Related Macular Degeneration and Retinitis Pigmentosa.

References

[1] http://education.yahoo.com/reference/gray/subjects/subject?id=225#p1016
[2] Cassin, B. and Solomon, S. (2001). *Dictionary of eye terminology.* Gainesville, Fla: Triad Pub. Co. ISBN 0-937404-63-2.
[3] Boyer MM, Poulsen GL, Nork TM. "Relative contributions of the neurosensory retina and retinal pigment epithelium to macular hypofluorescence." Arch Ophthalmol. 2000 Jan;118(1):27-31. PMID 10636410.
[4] Coscas, Gabriel and Felice Cardillo Piccolino (1998). *Retinal Pigment Epithelium and Macular Diseases.* Springer. ISBN 0792351444.
[5] "eye, human."Encyclopædia Britannica from Encyclopædia Britannica 2006 Ultimate Reference Suite DVD 2009

External links

- MeSH *pigment+epithelium+of+eye* (http://www.nlm.nih.gov/cgi/mesh/2011/MB_cgi?mode=& term=pigment+epithelium+of+eye)
- Histology at BU *07902loa* (http://www.bu.edu/histology/p/07902loa.htm)
- Histology at KUMC *eye_ear-eye11* (http://www.kumc.edu/instruction/medicine/anatomy/histoweb/eye_ear/ eye11.htm)

This article was originally based on an entry from a public domain edition of Gray's Anatomy. *As such, some of the information contained within it may be outdated.*

Retina

Retina	
Right human eye cross-sectional view. Courtesy NIH National Eye Institute. Many animals have eyes different from the human eye.	
Gray's	subject #225 1014 [1]
Artery	central retinal artery
MeSH	Retina [2]
Dorlands/Elsevier	Retina [3]

The vertebrate **retina** is a light-sensitive tissue lining the inner surface of the eye. The optics of the eye create an image of the visual world on the retina, which serves much the same function as the film in a camera. Light striking the retina initiates a cascade of chemical and electrical events that ultimately trigger nerve impulses. These are sent to various visual centers of the brain through the fibers of the optic nerve.

In vertebrate embryonic development, the retina and the optic nerve originate as outgrowths of the developing brain, so the retina is considered part of the central nervous system (CNS).[4] It is the only part of the CNS that can be visualized non-invasively.

The retina is a complex, layered structure with several layers of neurons interconnected by synapses. The only neurons that are directly sensitive to light are the photoreceptor cells. These are mainly of two types: the rods and cones. Rods function mainly in dim light and provide black-and-white vision, while cones support daytime vision and the perception of colour. A third, much rarer type of photoreceptor, the photosensitive ganglion cell, is important for reflexive responses to bright daylight.

Neural signals from the rods and cones undergo complex processing by other neurons of the retina. The output takes the form of action potentials in retinal ganglion cells whose axons form the optic nerve. Several important features of visual perception can be traced to the retinal encoding and processing of light.

Anatomy of vertebrate retina

The vertebrate retina has ten distinct layers.[5] From innermost to outermost, they include:

1. *Inner limiting membrane* – Müller cell footplates
2. *Nerve fiber layer* – essentially the axons of the ganglion cell nuclei
3. *Ganglion cell layer* – layer that contains nuclei of ganglion cells, the axons of which become the optic nerve fibers for messages[4]
4. *Inner plexiform layer* – contains the synapse between the bipolar cell axons and the dendrites of the ganglion and amacrine cells.[4]

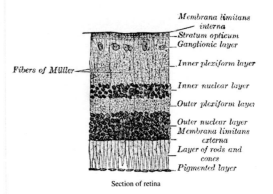

Section of retina

5. *Inner nuclear layer* – contains the nuclei and surrounding cell bodies (perikarya) of the bipolar cells, which correspond to heat and touch sensory skin receptors transmitting signals to the spinal cord or its continuation, the medulla.[4]
6. *Outer plexiform layer* – projections of rods and cones ending in the rod spherule and cone pedicle, respectively. These make synapses with dendrites of bipolar[4] In the macular region, this is known as the *Fiber layer of Henle.*
7. *Outer nuclear layer* –
8. *External limiting membrane* – layer that separates the inner segment portions of the photoreceptors from their cell nucleus
9. *Photoreceptor layer* – rods/cones
10. *Retinal pigment epithelium*

Of these the four main layers of the ten, from outside in: pigment epithelium, the photoreceptor layer for sight, bipolar cells, and finally, the ganglion cell layer which also contains photoreceptors, the photosensitive ganglion cells.

Therefore, the optic nerve is less a nerve than a central tract, connecting the bipolars to the lateral geniculate body, a visual relay station in the diencephalon (the rear of the forebrain).[4] Additional structures, not directly associated with vision, are found as outgrowths of the retina in some vertebrate groups. In birds, the pecten is a vascular structure of complex shape that projects from the retina into the vitreous humour; it supplies oxygen and nutrients to the eye, and may also aid in vision. Reptiles have a similar, but much simpler, structure, referred to as the *papillary cone.*[6]

Physical structure of human retina

In adult humans the entire retina is approximately 72% of a sphere about 22 mm in diameter. The entire retina contains about 7 million cones and 75 to 150 million rods. The optic disc, a part of the retina sometimes called "the blind spot" because it lacks photoreceptors, is located at the optic papilla, a nasal zone where the optic-nerve fibers leave the eye. It appears as an oval white area of 3mm². Temporal (in the direction of the temples) to this disc is the macula. At its center is the fovea, a pit that is responsible for our sharp central vision but is actually less sensitive to light because of its lack of rods. Human and non-human primates possess one fovea as opposed to certain bird species such as hawks who actually are bifoviate and dogs and cats who possess no fovea but a central band known as the visual streak. Around the fovea extends the central retina for about 6 mm and then the peripheral retina. The edge of the retina is defined by the ora serrata. The length from one ora to the other (or macula), the most sensitive area along the horizontal meridian is about 3.2 mm.

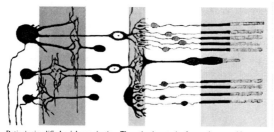

Retina's simplified axial organization. The retina is a stack of several neuronal layers. Light is concentrated from the eye and passes across these layers (from left to right) to hit the photoreceptors (right layer). This elicits chemical transformation mediating a propagation of signal to the bipolar and horizontal cells (middle yellow layer). The signal is then propagated to the amacrine and ganglion cells. These neurons ultimately may produce action potentials on their axons. This spatiotemporal pattern of spikes determines the raw input from the eyes to the brain. (Modified from a drawing by Ramón y Cajal.)

In section the retina is no more than 0.5 mm thick. It has three layers of nerve cells and two of synapses, including the unique ribbon synapses. The optic nerve carries the ganglion cell axons to the brain and the blood vessels that open into the retina. The ganglion cells lie innermost in the retina while the photoreceptive cells lie outermost. Because of this counter-intuitive arrangement, light must first pass through and around the ganglion cells and through the thickness of the retina, (including its capillary vessels, not shown) before reaching the rods and cones. However it does not pass through the epithelium or the choroid (both of which are opaque).

The white blood cells in the capillaries in front of the photoreceptors can be perceived as tiny bright moving dots when looking into blue light. This is known as the blue field entoptic phenomenon (or Scheerer's phenomenon).

Between the ganglion cell layer and the rods and cones there are two layers of neuropils where synaptic contacts are made. The neuropil layers are the outer plexiform layer and the inner plexiform layer. In the outer the rods and cones connect to the vertically running bipolar cells, and the horizontally oriented horizontal cells connect to ganglion cells.

The central retina is cone-dominated and the peripheral retina is rod-dominated. In total there are about seven million cones and a hundred million rods. At the centre of the macula is the foveal pit where the cones are smallest and in a hexagonal mosaic, the most efficient and highest density. Below the pit the other retina layers are displaced, before building up along the foveal slope until the rim of the fovea or parafovea which is the thickest portion of the retina. The macula has a yellow pigmentation from screening pigments and is known as the macula lutea. The area directly surrounding the fovea has the highest density of rods converging on single bipolars. Since the cones have a much lesser power of merging signals, the fovea allows for the sharpest vision the eye can attain.[4]

Though the rod and cones are a mosaic of sorts, transmission from receptors to bipolars to ganglion cells is not the case. Since there are about 150 million receptors and only 1 million optic nerve fibers, there must be convergence and thus mixing of signals. Moreover, the horizontal action of the horizontal and amacrine cells can allow one area of the retina to control another (e.g., one stimulus inhibiting another). This inhibition is key to the sum of messages sent to the higher regions of the brain. In some lower vertebrates, (e.g., the pigeon) there is a "centrifugal" control of messages, that is, one layer can control another, or higher regions of the brain can drive the retinal nerve cells, but in primates this does not occur.[4]

Vertebrate and cephalopod retina differences

The vertebrate retina is *inverted* in the sense that the light sensing cells sit at the back side of the retina, so that light has to pass through layers of neurons and capillaries before it reaches the rods and cones. By contrast, the cephalopod retina has the photoreceptors at the front side of the retina, with processing neurons and capillaries behind them. Because of this, cephalopods do not have a blind spot.

The cephalopod retina does not originate as an outgrowth of the brain, as the vertebrate one does. It was originally argued that this difference shows that vertebrate and cephalopod eyes are not homologous but have evolved separately. The evolutionary biologist Richard Dawkins cites the imperfect structure of the human retina as confounding claims by creationists or intelligent design theorists that the human eye is so perfect it must have a designer.[7]

In 2009 Kröger anatomically showed in Zebrafish that though the inverted arrangement is nonadaptive in that it creates avoidable scattering of light (and thus loss of light and image blur), it has space-saving advantages for small-eyed animals in which there is a minimal vitreous body, as the space between the lens and the photoreceptors' light-sensitive outer segments is completely filled with retinal cells.[8]

Physiology

An image is produced by the patterned excitation of the cones and rods in the retina. The excitation is processed by the neuronal system and various parts of the brain working in parallel to form a representation of the external environment in the brain.

The cones respond to bright light and mediate high-resolution colour vision during daylight illumination (also called photopic vision). The rods are saturated at daylight levels and don't contribute to pattern vision. However, rods do respond to dim light and mediate lower-resolution, monochromatic vision under very low levels of illumination (called scotopic vision). The illumination in most office settings falls between these two levels and is called mesopic vision. At these light levels, both the rods and cones are actively contributing pattern information to that exiting the eye. What contribution the rod information makes to pattern vision under these circumstances is unclear.

The response of cones to various wavelengths of light is called their spectral sensitivity. In normal human vision, the spectral sensitivity of a cone falls into one of three subgroups. These are often called red, green, and blue cones but more accurately are short, medium, and long wavelength sensitive cone subgroups. It is a lack of one or more of the cone subtypes that causes individuals to have deficiencies in colour vision or various kinds of colour blindness. These individuals are not blind to objects of a particular colour but experience the inability to distinguish between two groups of colours that *can* be distinguished by people with normal vision. Humans have three different types of cones (trichromatic vision) while most other mammals lack cones with red sensitive pigment and therefore have poorer (dichromatic) colour vision. However, some animals have four spectral subgroups, e.g., the trout adds an ultraviolet subgroup to short, medium and long subgroups that are similar to humans. Some fish are sensitive to the polarization of light as well.

When light falls on a receptor it sends a proportional response synaptically to bipolar cells which in turn signal the retinal ganglion cells. The receptors are also 'cross-linked' by horizontal cells and amacrine cells, which modify the synaptic signal before the ganglion cells. Rod and cone signals are intermixed and combine, although rods are mostly active in very poorly lit conditions and saturate in broad daylight, while cones function in brighter lighting because they are not sensitive enough to work at very low light levels.

Despite the fact that all are nerve cells, only the retinal ganglion cells and few amacrine cells create action potentials. In the photoreceptors, exposure to light hyperpolarizes the membrane in a series of graded shifts. The outer cell segment contains a photopigment. Inside the cell the normal levels of cyclic guanosine monophosphate (cGMP) keep the Na+ channel open and thus in the resting state the cell is depolarised. The photon causes the retinal bound to the receptor protein to isomerise to trans-retinal. This causes receptor to activate multiple G-proteins. This in turn causes the Ga-subunit of the protein to bind and degrade cGMP inside the cell which then cannot bind to the Na+ cyclic nucleotide-gated ion channels (CNGs). Thus the cell is hyperpolarised. The amount of neurotransmitter released is reduced in bright light and increases as light levels fall. The actual photopigment is bleached away in bright light and only replaced as a chemical process, so in a transition from bright light to darkness the eye can take up to thirty minutes to reach full sensitivity (see Adaptation (eye)).

In the retinal ganglion cells there are two types of response, depending on the receptive field of the cell. The receptive fields of retinal ganglion cells comprise a central approximately circular area, where light has one effect on the firing of the cell, and an annular surround, where light has the opposite effect on the firing of the cell. In ON cells, an increment in light intensity in the centre of the receptive field causes the firing rate to increase. In OFF cells, it makes it decrease. In a linear model, this response profile is well described by a Difference of Gaussians and is the basis for edge detection algorithms. Beyond this simple difference ganglion cells are also differentiated by chromatic sensitivity and the type of spatial summation. Cells showing linear spatial summation are termed X cells (also called parvocellular, P, or midget ganglion cells), and those showing non-linear summation are Y cells (also called magnocellular, M, or parasol retinal ganglion cells), although the correspondence between X and Y cells (in the cat retina) and P and M cells (in the primate retina) is not as simple as it once seemed.

In the transfer of visual signals to the brain, the visual pathway, the retina is vertically divided in two, a temporal (nearer to the temple) half and a nasal (nearer to the nose) half. The axons from the nasal half cross the brain at the optic chiasma to join with axons from the temporal half of the other eye before passing into the lateral geniculate body.

Although there are more than 130 million retinal receptors, there are only approximately 1.2 million fibres (axons) in the optic nerve; a large amount of pre-processing is performed within the retina. The fovea produces the most accurate information. Despite occupying about 0.01% of the visual field (less than 2° of visual angle), about 10% of axons in the optic nerve are devoted to the fovea. The resolution limit of the fovea has been determined at around 10,000 points. The information capacity is estimated at 500,000 bits per second (for more information on bits, see information theory) without colour or around 600,000 bits per second including colour.

Spatial encoding

The retina, unlike a camera, does not simply send a picture to the brain. The retina spatially encodes (compresses) the image to fit the limited capacity of the optic nerve. Compression is necessary because there are 100 times more Photoreceptor cells than ganglion cells as mentioned above. The retina does so by "decorrelating" the incoming images in a manner to be described below. These operations are carried out by the center surround structures as implemented by the bipolar and ganglion cells.

There are two types of center surround structures in the retina—on-centers and off-centers. On-centers have a positively weighted center and a negatively weighted surround. Off-centers are just the opposite. Positive weighting is more commonly known as excitatory and negative weighting is more commonly known as inhibitory.

These center surround structures are not physical in the sense that you cannot see them by staining samples of tissue and examining the retina's anatomy. The center surround structures are logical (i.e., mathematically abstract) in the sense that they depend on the connection strengths between ganglion and bipolar cells. It is believed that the connection strengths between cells is caused by the number and types of ion channels embedded in the synapses between the ganglion and bipolar cells. Stephen Kuffler in the 1950s was the first person to begin to understand these center surround structures in the retina of cats. See Receptive field for figures and more information on center surround structures. See chapter 3 of David Hubel's on-line book (listed below) for an excellent introduction.

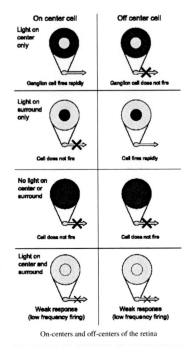

On-centers and off-centers of the retina

The center surround structures are mathematically equivalent to the edge detection algorithms used by computer programmers to extract or enhance the edges in a digital photograph. Thus the retina performs operations on the image to enhance the edges of objects within its visual field. For example, in a picture of a dog, a cat and a car, it is the edges of these objects that contain the most information. In order for higher functions in the brain (or in a computer for that matter) to extract and classify objects such as a dog and a cat, the retina is the first step to separating out the various objects within the scene.

As an example, the following matrix is at the heart of the computer algorithm that implements edge detection. This matrix is the computer equivalent to the center surround structure. In this example, each box (element) within this matrix would be connected to one photoreceptor. The photoreceptor in the center is the current receptor being processed. The center photoreceptor is multiplied by the +1 weight factor. The surrounding photoreceptors are the "nearest neighbors" to the center and are multiplied by the -1/8 value. The sum of all nine of these elements is finally calculated. This summation is repeated for every photoreceptor in the image by shifting left to the end of a row and then down to the next line.

-1/8	-1/8	-1/8
-1/8	+1	-1/8
-1/8	-1/8	-1/8

The total sum of this matrix is zero if all the inputs from the nine photoreceptors are the same value. The zero result indicates the image was uniform (non-changing) within this small patch. Negative or positive sums mean something was varying (changing) within this small patch of nine photoreceptors.

The above matrix is only an approximation to what really happens inside the retina. The differences are:

1. The above example is called "balanced". The term balanced means that the sum of the negative weights is equal to the sum of the positive weights so that they cancel out perfectly. Retinal ganglion cells are almost never perfectly balanced.

2. The table is square while the center surround structures in the retina are circular.

3. Neurons operate on spike trains traveling down nerve cell axons. Computers operate on a single Floating point number that is essentially constant from each input pixel. (The computer pixel is basically the equivalent of a biological photoreceptor.)

4. The retina performs all these calculations in parallel while the computer operates on each pixel one at a time. There are no repeated summations and shifting as there would be in a computer.

5. Finally, the horizontal and amacrine cells play a significant role in this process but that is not represented here.

Here is an example of an input image and how edge detection would modify it.

Input Image – Original At Photoreceptors		Output Image – Compressed Traveling down axons of Ganglion Cells

Ultra Black Font ⟶ Retina ⟶ Ultra Black Font

Once the image is spatially encoded by the center surround structures, the signal is sent out the optical nerve (via the axons of the ganglion cells) through the optic chiasm to the LGN (lateral geniculate nucleus). The exact function of the LGN is unknown at this time. The output of the LGN is then sent to the back of the brain. Specifically the output of the LGN "radiates" out to the V1 Primary visual cortex.

Simplified Signal Flow: Photoreceptors → Bipolar → Ganglion → Chiasm → LGN → V1 cortex

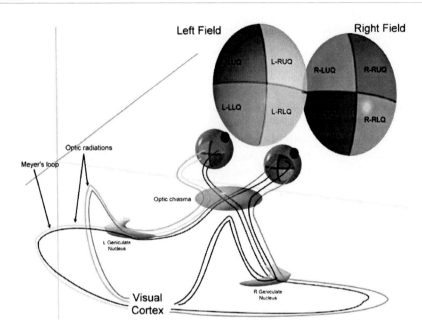

Diseases and disorders

There are many inherited and acquired diseases or disorders that may affect the retina. Some of them include:

- Retinitis pigmentosa is a group of genetic diseases that affect the retina and causes the loss of night vision and peripheral vision.
- Macular degeneration describes a group of diseases characterized by loss of central vision because of death or impairment of the cells in the macula.
- Cone-rod dystrophy (CORD) describes a number of diseases where vision loss is caused by deterioration of the cones and/or rods in the retina.
- In retinal separation, the retina detaches from the back of the eyeball. Ignipuncture is an outdated treatment method. The term retinal detachment is used to describe a separation of the neurosensory retina from the retinal pigment epithelium.[9] There are several modern treatment methods for fixing a retinal detachment: pneumatic retinopexy, scleral buckle, cryotherapy, laser photocoagulation and pars plana vitrectomy.
- Both hypertension and diabetes mellitus can cause damage to the tiny blood vessels that supply the retina, leading to hypertensive retinopathy and diabetic retinopathy.
- Retinoblastoma is a cancer of the retina.
- Retinal diseases in dogs include retinal dysplasia, progressive retinal atrophy, and sudden acquired retinal degeneration.
- *Lipemia retinalis* is a white appearance of the retina, and can occur by lipid deposition in lipoprotein lipase deficiency.

Diagnosis and treatment

A number of different instruments are available for the diagnosis of diseases and disorders affecting the retina. An ophthalmoscope is used to examine the retina. Recently, adaptive optics has been used to image individual rods and cones in the living human retina and a company based in Scotland have engineered technology that allows physicians to observe the complete retina without any discomfort to patients.[10] The electroretinogram is used to measure non-invasively the retina's electrical activity, which is affected by certain diseases. A relatively new technology, now becoming widely available, is optical coherence tomography (OCT). This non-invasive technique allows one to obtain a 3D volumetric or high resolution cross-sectional tomogram of the retinal fine structure with histologic-quality.

Treatment depends upon the nature of the disease or disorder. Transplantation of retinas has been attempted, but without much success. At MIT, The University of Southern California, and the University of New South Wales, an "artificial retina" is under development: an implant which will bypass the photoreceptors of the retina and stimulate the attached nerve cells directly, with signals from a digital camera.

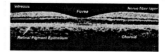

OCT scan of a retina at 800nm with an axial resolution of 3μm

Retinal blood supply

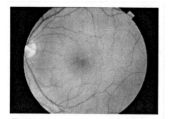

The blood vessels in a normal human retina. The optic disk is at extreme left, and the macula lutea is near the center.

There are two circulations, both supplied by the ophthalmic artery. The uveal circulation consists of arteries entering the globe outside the optic nerve, these supply the uvea and outer and middle layers of the retina. The retinal circulation, on the other hand, supplies the inner layer of the retina and passes with the optic nerve as a branch of the ophthalmic artery called the central artery of the retina.[4] The unique structure of the blood vessels in the retina has been used for biometric identification.

Research

George Wald, Haldan Keffer Hartline and Ragnar Granit won the 1967 Nobel Prize in Physiology or Medicine for their scientific research on the retina.

A recent University of Pennsylvania study calculated the approximate bandwidth of human retinas is 8.75 megabits per second, whereas guinea pig retinas transfer at 875 kilobits.[11]

MacLaren & Pearson and colleagues at University College London and Moorfields Eye Hospital in London showed in 2006 that photoreceptor cells could be transplanted successfully in the mouse retina if donor cells were at a critical developmental stage.[12] Recently Ader and colleagues in Dublin showed using the electron microscope that transplanted photoreceptors formed synaptic connections.[13]

Retinal gene therapy

Gene therapy holds promise as a potential avenue to cure a wide range of retinal diseases. This involves using a non-infectious virus to shuttle a gene into a part of the retina. Recombinant adeno-associated virus (rAAV) vectors possess a number of features that render them ideally suited for retinal gene therapy, including a lack of pathogenicity, minimal immunogenicity, and the ability to transduce postmitotic cells in a stable and efficient manner.[14] rAAV vectors are increasingly utilized for their ability to mediate efficient transduction of retinal pigment epithelium (RPE), photoreceptor cells and retinal ganglion cells. Each cell type can be specifically targeted by choosing the appropriate combination of AAV serotype, promoter, and intraocular injection site.

The unique architecture of the retina and its relatively immune-privileged environment help this process. Tight junctions that form the blood retinal barrier separate the subretinal space from the blood supply, thus protecting it from microbes and most immune-mediated damage, and enhancing its potential to respond to vector-mediated therapies. The highly compartmentalized anatomy of the eye facilitates accurate delivery of therapeutic vector suspensions to specific tissues under direct visualization using microsurgical techniques.[15] In the sheltered environment of the retina, AAV vectors are able to maintain high levels of transgene expression in the retinal pigmented epithelium (RPE), photoreceptors, or ganglion cells for long periods of time after a single treatment. In addition, the eye and the visual system can be routinely and easily monitored for visual function and retinal structural changes after injections with noninvasive advanced technology, such as visual acuities, contrast sensitivity, fundus auto-fluorescence (FAF), dark-adapted visual thresholds, vascular diameters, pupillometry, electroretinography (ERG), multifocal ERG and optical coherence tomography (OCT).[16]

This strategy is effective against retinal diseases that have been studied including neovascular diseases that are features of age-related macular degeneration, diabetic retinopathy and retinopathy of prematurity. Since the regulation of vascularization in the mature retina involves a balance between endogenous positive growth factors, such as vascular endothelial growth factor (VEGF) and inhibitors of angiogenesis, such as pigment epithelium-derived factor (PEDF), rAAV-mediated expression of PEDF, angiostatin, and the soluble VEGF receptor sFlt-1, which are all antiangiogenic proteins, have been shown to reduce aberrant vessel formation in animal models.[17] Since specific gene therapies cannot readily be used to treat a significant fraction of patients with retinal dystrophy, there is a major interest in developing a more generally applicable survival factor therapy. Neurotrophic factors have the ability to modulate neuronal growth during development to maintain existing cells and to allow recovery of injured neuronal populations in the eye. AAV encoding neurotrophic factors such as fibroblast growth factor (FGF) family members and GDNF either protected photoreceptors from apoptosis or slowed down cell death.[17]

However, treatment of inherited retinal degenerative diseases such as retinitis pigmentosa and Leber congenital amaurosis (LCA) via gene replacement therapy constitutes the most straightforward and therefore the most promising approach for treating the autosomal recessive retinal disease. Leber Congenital Amaurosis (LCA2) is a defect of the *RPE65* gene, which is responsible for the synthesis of 11-cis retinal, an important molecule in the visual phototransduction, and gene replacement therapy studies utilizing *rpe65*-encoding AAV have yielded hopeful results in animal models.[18] Based on several encouraging reports from animal models, at least three clinical trials are currently underway for the treatment of LCA using modified AAV vectors carrying the RPE65 cDNA and have reported positive preliminary results.[19]

References

[1] http://education.yahoo.com/reference/gray/subjects/subject?id=225#p1014

[2] http://www.nlm.nih.gov/cgi/mesh/2007/MB_cgi?mode=&term=Retina

[3] http://www.mercksource.com/pp/us/cns/cns_hl_dorlands_split.jsp?pg=/ppdocs/us/common/dorlands/dorland/seven/000092489.htm

[4] "Sensory Reception: Human Vision: Structure and functioon of the Human Eye" vol. 27, Encyclopaedia Britannica, 1987

[5] The Retinal Tunic (http://education.vetmed.vt.edu/Curriculum/VM8054/EYE/RETINA.HTM)

[6] Romer, Alfred Sherwood; Parsons, Thomas S. (1977). *The Vertebrate Body*. Philadelphia, PA: Holt-Saunders International. p. 465. ISBN 0-03-910284-X.

[7] Dawkins, Richard (1986). *The Blind Watchmaker*. Longman. p. 93. ISBN 0-582-44694-5. "An engineer would laugh at any suggestion that the photocells might point away from the light, with their wires departing on the side *nearest* the light. Yet this is what happens in all vertebrate retinas. The wire has to travel over the surface of the retina to a point where it dives through a hole in the retina, (the so-called blind spot) to joint the optic nerve. Light..has to pass through a forest of connecting wires, presumably suffering at least some attenuation and distortion....the principle of the thing would offend any tidy-minded engineer"

[8] Kröger RH, Biehlmaier O. (2009). Space saving advantage of an inverted retina. Vision Res. 49(18):2318-21. PMID 19591859

[9] Oh, Kean, "Pathogenetic Mechanisms of Retinal Detachment", in Retina, ed. Ryan, S.J., Elsevier Health Sciences, Philadelphia, PA, 2006, p. 2013-2015

[10] Seeing into the Future (http://www.ingenia.org.uk/ingenia/articles.aspx?Index=414) *Ingenia*, March 2007

[11] Calculating the speed of sight - being-human - 28 July 2006 - New Scientist (http://www.newscientist.com/article/dn9633-calculating-the-speed-of-sight.html)

[12] Retinal repair by transplantation of photoreceptor precursors : Abstract : Nature (http://www.nature.com/nature/journal/v444/n7116/abs/nature05161.html)

[13] Retinal cells integrate into the outer nuclear layer and differentiate into mature photoreceptors after subretinal transplantation into adult mice (http://www.ncbi.nlm.nih.gov/pubmed/18329018)

[14] Astra Dinculescu, Lyudmyla Glushakova, Seok-Hong Min, William W. Hauswirth. *Human Gene Therapy*. June 2005, 16(6): 649-663.

[15] Enrico M. Curace, Alberto Auricchio. Versatility of AAV vectors for retinal gene transfer. *Vision Research*. 2008, 48:353-359.

[16] Anneke I. den Hollandera, Ronald Roepmana, Robert K. Koenekoopb, Frans P.M. Cremersa. Leber congenital amaurosis: Genes, proteins and disease mechanisms. *Progress in Retinal and Eye Research*. July 2008; 27(4):391-419.

[17] Rolling F. Recombinant AAV-mediated gene transfer to the retina: gene therapy perspectives. *Gene Therapy*. 2004; 11: S26-S32.

[18] Tonia S. Rex. Rescue of Sight by Gene Therapy − Closer than It May Appear. *Ophthalmic Genetics*. 2007, 28:127-133.

[19] Xue Cai, Shannon M. Conley, Muna I Naash. RPE65: Role in the Visual Cycle, Human Retinal Disease, and Gene Therapy. *Ophthalmic Genetics*. June 2009, 30(2):57-62.

Further reading

- S. Ramón y Cajal, *Histologie du Système Nerveux de l'Homme et des Vertébrés*, Maloine, Paris, 1911.
- Rodieck RW (1965). "Quantitative analysis of cat retinal ganglion cell response to visual stimuli". *Vision Res.* 5 (11): 583–601. doi:10.1016/0042-6989(65)90033-7. PMID 5862581.
- Wandell, Brian A. (1995). *Foundations of vision*. Sunderland, Mass: Sinauer Associates. ISBN 0-87893-853-2.
- Wässle H, Boycott BB (1991). "Functional architecture of the mammalian retina". *Physiol Rev.* 71 (2): 447–480. PMID 2006220.
- Schulz HL, Goetz T, Kaschkoetoe J, Weber BH (2004). "The Retinome - defining a reference transcriptome of the adult mammalian retina/retinal pigment epithelium" (http://www.pubmedcentral.nih.gov/articlerender.fcgi?tool=pmcentrez&artid=512282). *BMC Genomics* 5 (1): 50. doi:10.1186/1471-2164-5-50. PMID 15283859. PMC 512282.

External links

- Eye, Brain, and Vision - online book - by David Hubel (http://neuro.med.harvard.edu/site/dh/index.html)
- Kolb, H., Fernandez, E., & Nelson, R. (2003). The neural organization of the vertebrate retina (http://webvision.med.utah.edu). Salt Lake City, Utah: John Moran Eye Center, University of Utah. Retrieved July 19, 2004.
- Demo: Artificial Retina (http://www.techreview.com/articles/04/09/demo0904.asp), MIT Technology Review, September 2004. Reports on implant research at Technology Review
- Successful photoreceptor transplantation (http://www.technologyreview.com/Biotech/17768), MIT Technology Review, November 2006. How stem cells might restore sight Technology Review
- Australian Vision Prosthesis Group (http://bionic.gsbme.unsw.edu.au/), Graduate School of Biomedical Engineering, University of New South Wales
- RetinaCentral (http://www.retinacentral.org), Genetics and Diseases of the Human Retina at University of Würzburg
- Retinal layers image. (http://www.ncbi.nlm.nih.gov/books/bv.fcgi?rid=neurosci.figgrp.740) NeuroScience 2nd Ed at United States National Library of Medicine
- The Vertebrate Retina: Structure, Function, and Evolution (http://ascb.org/ibioseminars/Nathans/nathans1a.cfm) on-line lecture by Jeremy Nathans
- Retina - Cell Centered Database (http://ccdb.ucsd.edu/sand/main?mpid=54&event=displaySum)
- Histology at BU *07901loa* (http://www.bu.edu/histology/p/07901loa.htm)

Peripheral vision

Peripheral vision is a part of vision that occurs outside the very center of gaze. There is a broad set of non-central points in the field of view that is included in the notion of peripheral vision. "Far peripheral" vision exists at the edges of the field of view, "mid-peripheral" vision exists in the middle of the field of view, and "near-peripheral", sometimes referred to as "para-central" vision, exists adjacent to the center of gaze.

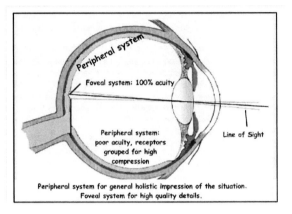

Peripheral system for general holistic impression of the situation. Foveal system for high quality details.

The loss of peripheral vision while retaining central vision is known as tunnel vision, and the loss of central vision while retaining peripheral vision is known as central scotoma.

Peripheral vision is weaker in humans, compared with other animals, especially at distinguishing color and shape. This is because receptor cells on the retina are greater at the center and lowest at the edges (see visual system for an explanation of these concepts). In addition, there are two types of receptor cells, rod cells and cone cells; rod cells are unable to distinguish color and are predominant at the periphery, while cone cells are concentrated mostly in the center of the retina, the fovea.

Flicker fusion threshold is higher for peripheral than foveal vision. Peripheral vision is good at detecting motion (a feature of rod cells).

Peripheral vision is hard to study in an objective manner, because there is no way to separate the visual detection of the eye from the neural processing of the brain. While the eye can be dissected and examined under a microscope, even if the entirety of the retina is capable of detecting light, that capacity may not be fully utilized or may not be consciously aware within the brain. Certain conditions such as lazy eye can cause suppression of an otherwise usable visual field, while stroke or damage to the corpus callosum can prevent left/right integration.

It is not possible to directly observe what the brain is detecting and comprehending, so research primarily involves perception tests based on reactions of test subjects to simulated stimuli. This testing is commonly carried out by requesting test subjects to focus on an object in front of them and then flashing lights at increasing distances away from the center of the visual field, noting the subject's reactions.

Central vision is relatively weak at night or in the dark, when the lack of color cues and lighting makes cone cells far less useful. Rod cells, which are concentrated further away from the retina, operate better than cone cells in low light. This makes peripheral vision useful for seeing movement at night. In fact, pilots are taught to use peripheral vision to scan for aircraft at night.

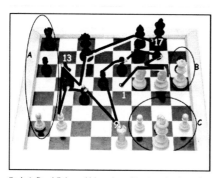

Ovals A, B and C show which portions of the chess situation a chess master can reproduce correctly with his peripheral vision. Lines show path of foveal fixation during 5 seconds when the task is to memorize the situation as correctly as possible. Image from [1] based on data by [2]

The distinctions between foveal (sometimes also called central) and peripheral vision are reflected in subtle physiological and anatomical differences in the visual cortex. Different visual areas contribute to the processing of visual information coming from different parts of the visual field, and a complex of visual areas located along the banks of the interhemispheric fissure (a deep groove that separates the two brain hemispheres) has been linked to peripheral vision. It has been suggested that these areas are important for fast reactions to visual stimuli in the periphery, and monitoring body position relative to gravity.[3]

Peripheral vision can be practiced, jugglers that regularly locate and catch objects in their peripheral vision do have improved abilities. Jugglers do not follow the paths of individual objects with their eyes, instead they focus on a defined point in mid-air, so almost all of the information necessary for successful catches is perceived in the near-peripheral region. Some juggling patterns and disciplines require extraordinary peripheral vision.

Being fully aware of your peripheral vision allows you to focus on your entire field of vision instead of focusing on just one spot. This should enable you to notice small movements at the edge of your sight and so be more aware of your surroundings and ready to react to things other than those directly in front of you. The opening move from the Karate form 'Kushan Ku' includes a move used to quickly engage peripheral vision. Standing with your hands hanging down in front, palms facing inward (one hand on top of the other), you then raise them directly in front of yourself so that you are pointing at the sky and they are at the top of your field of vision. While still looking forward, but concentrating on seeing your hands, you then bring them down by either side, slowly drawing a large circle and ending up in the starting position but with your palms facing outward. As they come down you should follow them without moving your gaze and so becoming fully aware of the area inside the circle.[4]

Functions

The main functions of peripheral vision are[1] :

- recognition of well-known structures and forms with no need to focus by the foveal line of sight.
- identification of similar forms and movements (Gestalt psychology laws)
- delivery of sensations which form the background of detailed visual perception.

References

[1] Hans-Werner Hunziker, (2006) Im Auge des Lesers: foveale und periphere Wahrnehmung - vom Buchstabieren zur Lesefreude [In the eye of the reader: foveal and peripheral perception - from letter recognition to the joy of reading] Transmedia Stäubli Verlag Zürich 2006 ISBN 978-3-7266-0068-6

[2] DE GROOT, A. : Perception and memory in chess; an experimental study of the heuristics of the professional eye. Mimeograph; Psychologisch Laboratorium Universiteit van Amsterdam, Seminarium September 1969

[3] Palmer SM, Rosa MG (2006). "A distinct anatomical network of cortical areas for analysis of motion in far peripheral vision". Eur J Neurosci 24 (8): 2389–405. doi:10.1111/j.1460-9568.2006.05113.x. PMID 17042793.

[4] http://www.betterhumans.com/blogs/squirrel_monkey/archive/2008/09/01/Improve-your-senses.aspx

Degenerative disease

A **degenerative disease**, also called neurodegenerative disease, is a disease in which the function or structure of the affected tissues or organs will progressively deteriorate over time, whether due to normal bodily wear or lifestyle choices such as exercise or eating habits.[1] Degenerative diseases are often contrasted with infectious diseases.

Some Examples of Degenerative Diseases

- Amyotrophic Lateral Sclerosis (ALS), e.g., Lou Gehrig's Disease
- Alzheimer's disease
- Parkinson's Disease
- Multiple system atrophy
- Niemann Pick disease
- Atherosclerosis
- Progressive supranuclear palsy
- Cancer
- Tay-Sachs Disease
- Diabetes
- Heart Disease
- Keratoconus
- Inflammatory Bowel Disease (IBD)
- Prostatitis
- Osteoarthritis
- Osteoporosis
- Rheumatoid Arthritis
- Huntington's Disease
- Chronic traumatic encephalopathy

References

[1] Degenerative Nerve Diseases (http://www.nlm.nih.gov/medlineplus/degenerativenervediseases.html)

Article Sources and Contributors

Retinitis pigmentosa *Source*: http://en.wikipedia.org/w/index.php?oldid=412307349 *Contributors*: 5 albert square, AED, Aggarsandeep, Alansohn, Alexius08, Altenmann, Arcadian, Arenmk1, Arhant, Axl, BWJones, Belinrahs, Beyond My Ken, BigGuy, Binarypascal, Boghog, Cg770, ClockworkSoul, ColorOfSuffering, CopperKettle, Coulraphobic123, Ctbolt, Daisy3211420, Danni09, Deelite72, Docu, Dougher, Dpryan, Drbreznjev, Dreslough, Dunhere, EoGuy, Erielhonan, Esparkhu, Falcon8765, Fama Clamosa, Farside, Filzstift, G716, Gigstars, GrahamDo, Grika, Gökhan, Herbee, Hordaland, Horologium, Ilyanep, Inchwell, J 1982, J04n, JamesAM, Jamesday, Jamocaha, Jevansen, Jharris0221, Joelmills, John of Reading, Katarinas, KrakatoaKatie, Lipothymia, Lisatwo, MK8, Mannerssarah, MaureensMenagerie, Max rspct, Maximus Rex, Mcrech1111, Msh210, NancySolari, NawlinWiki, Nikiscool, Niranjanpalvankar, Nono64, Oboeboy, Oghmoir, Patenaude, Paul venter, Piksteel, Prosfilaes, RDBrown, Rchaud2, Rdrozd, Reyk, Rich Farmbrough, Richerman, Rjwilmsi, Roberta F., Robomojo, Rod57, Ronz, Rpinternational1972, Rumsdoc, SJHL100, Sagaciousuk, Sarrus, Scottalter, Shehperpk, Skittleys, Snagglepuss, Solipsist, Spaceanddeath, Spitfire, Stone, T J McKenzie, Tassedethe, Tharold, TheoldGP, Tofutwitch11, ToobMug, Trachtemacht, Tuur, Ved Prakash Banga, Vicki Rosenzweig, Woohookitty, Wouterstomp, Yer maw, Ævar Arnfjörð Bjarmason, 189 anonymous edits

Human eye *Source*: http://en.wikipedia.org/w/index.php?oldid=412659639 *Contributors*: 1111mol, 5 albert square, A302b, Ahpook, Aks06, Alansohn, Alexsamson, Alkasi2000, Antandrus, Arancaytar, Arcadian, Asdofindia, Ash, Assianir, Autumnwashere, BDD88 59 9, Barek, Beland, Bengish, Berichard, Beyond My Ken, Bomber62, C6H3N3O3, CMG, Casseck, Chasingsol, Chizeng, Chowbok, Cindyswu, Ckatz, Cliff smith, CliffC, Courcelles, Cpl Syx, DARTH SIDIOUS 2, Darkwind, Dave3457, Dbfirs, Dontshootjimmy, Duncan, Elassint, Epastore, Epbr123, Esoteric Rogue, Eve Hall, Excirial, Fama Clamosa, Furado, Fyyer, Garrettaggs55, Gary King, Gfoley4, Ghogg, Hertz1888, Hordaland, Immunize, Imnotminkus, Ingolfson, J.delanoy, JNW, JOSamsung, Jabranafique, Jd Tendril, Jeff G., Jenneca07, JohnCD, JuhkoDev, Jusdafax, Kmoksy, Kristiani95, Kubigula, Leuko, Loupeter, Mannafredo, Matt Deres, Medtopic, Mild Bill Hiccup, Mohamed Osama AlNagdy, MoiraMoira, Monterey Bay, Newone, NickCT, Nk, Nono64, Nuvitauy07, Outback the koala, PMG, Peatswift, Pedgi, Petrb, Philip Trueman, Psychonaught, Quibik, Quintus314, RainbowDogSpecies, RayJohnstone, Realm of Shadows, Reaper Eternal, RetiredUser2, Rjwilmsi, Roberta F., Ronhjones, Rrburke, SF007, SURIV, Sand village, Scriberius, Sego Lily, Shadowjams, Shura007, Skatebiker, Smith609, Snigbrook, SpaceFlight89, Sparrer, Srleffler, Stormbreaker200, Tempodivalse, The High Fin Sperm Whale, Tide rolls, Tim bates, Tim010987, Tommy2010, V2Blast, Vlarfa, Woohookitty, World, Wtmitchell, XxDestinyxX, YH1975, 242 anonymous edits

Nyctalopia *Source*: http://en.wikipedia.org/w/index.php?oldid=409333078 *Contributors*: AED, AgentPeppermint, Ahoerstemeier, AkvoD3, Andjam, Antibaro, Arcadian, AsS30, BraneJ, Bubba hotep, Camw, Cendare, Christina121, CiaPan, Cooner750, CopperKettle, Crystallina, Cybercobra, Cyrius, Deli nk, DiogenesTCP, Enguehard, Famizban, Future Perfect at Sunrise, Gadfium, Gilliam, Gogo Dodo, Graevemoore, Grendelkhan, Gyurika, JRSP, Jemfinch, Johantheghost, JonnieZG, Josh Parris, Kandar, Katharinearny, Kjramesh, KlaudiuMihaila, KnightRider, LOL., Ligulem, LittleOldMe, Males, MarSch, Marora123, Meursault2004, Mikael Häggström, Mike Serfas, Montanabw, Mwanner, Nikuda, Nivedit Mishra, Pathless, Paul venter, Phils, Pion, Rfts, Scottalter, Shafei, Supine, TrackMonkey, Tuur, Urhixidur, VMS Mosaic, Vsmaverick, Wccaccamise, Whitepaw, William charles caccamise sr, md, זרם, 76 anonymous edits

Tunnel vision *Source*: http://en.wikipedia.org/w/index.php?oldid=408165385 *Contributors*: 100110100, AED, Aiko, Angela, Apteva, Azumanga1, BinaryTed, Blahma, Boffy b, Bornhj, Butros, CPAM, CrookedAsterisk, DMahafko, DabMachine, Discospinster, Eeblefish, Ex nihil, EyeMD, Folajimi, Formeruser-81, Gary King, Goatasaur, Gonzonoir, Gwjenkins, Hooperbloob, Jamesday, Johan Lont, JuJube, Kwertii, Kz9dsr0t387346, Lilbama, Lo2u, Lova Falk, Monkeyblue, Mordicai, OlEnglish, Orphan Wiki, Paul venter, Philip Trueman, PierreAbbat, Pinethicket, Raabusmc, Radagast83, Regano, Shadowjams, Shandris, Spindled, TGOO, The Anome, Timwi, Tobyr21, Ufinne, Viajero, Westbender, Wolfkeeper, 62 anonymous edits

Blindness *Source*: http://en.wikipedia.org/w/index.php?oldid=411505575 *Contributors*: 146.227.71.xxx, 16@r, 2D, ABF, AED, AJR, Aaron Schulz, Aaron Simon, Academic Challenger, AgainErick, AgentFade2Black, AgentPeppermint, Ahoerstemeier, Aikido man, Aitias, Ajsh, Akatimr, Akerans, Alansohn, Alessandro 10, Alex muller, Alex.tan, Algae, Algocu, AlistairMcMillan, Allstarecho, Altenmann, AnakngAraw, Andy M. Wang, Andycjp, Angela, Anonymous editor, Anthony Appleyard, Anthonyhcole, Aranel, Arcadian, Aramm88, Atlant, Axekiller1212, Barf012, Bart133, Beland, Belovedfreak, Benmelman, Bentley4, Betakate, Bhugh, BiT, Bib, Binky The WonderSkull, Bjbonewell, BlueDevil, BobbyMoinahan, Bobo192, Bonadea, Bowlhover, Brighteorange, Brinticus, Bryan Derksen, Bulldog333333333, BurgererSF, CERminator, CHILighthouse, CMat, CTZMSC3, Cabias, CambridgeBayWeather, Cameltrader, Camr, Canderson7, Captain panda, Captain-n00dle, CardinalDan, Cctoide, Cheejo, Cheymac, Chocolateboy, Chun-hian, ClockworkSoul, Conversion script, Cowpepper, Cryme-time, Cvaneg, Cyanoa Crylate, DVD R W, Dainsleif, Danceswithzerglings, Danzella, Darth Panda, Darthbob100, Dave treuman, Dave6, Dcreemer, December21st2012Freak, Dekisugi, Delirium, Delldot, Denni, Dialectric, Dictionary199, Diddlyman2004, Discospinster, Dlohcierekim, Dlrohrer2003, Doczilla, DolphinL, Dreadfullyboring, Dysprosia, E. Ripley, EEMIV, EaglePride5, EamonnPKeane, Edburke317, Edison, Edward, Efneal, Elijahg0, Ellywa, Emijrp, Enric Naval, Epbr123, Esmito, Essam Sharaf, Etoile, Eubulides, Ewlyahoocom, Excirial, Exeunt, Eyalshalom, EyeMD, F16, FF2010, FT2, Fabrictramp, Fang Aili, Faradayplank, Fedfefretfrgfeqrg, FisherQueen, Fishl, Florentino floro, Fredrik, FreplySpang, Frosted14, Furrykef, GRuban, Gabspeck, Gadfium, Gaius Cornelius, Garion96, George100, Gerstman ny, Giedrius S., Gilliam, Glenncomti, Gogo Dodo, GoldDragon, GorillaWarfare, Gothica36, Graham87, Gurubrahma, Gökhan, Hadal, HaeB, Haemo, Haham hanuka, Hariva, Harisd5917, Hawaiian717, Hbackman, Heathamanda, Hede2000, HelpingMind, HenryLi, Heron, HexaChord, Hey jude, don't let me down, HiLo FastSlow, HolIgor, Hordaland, Huyvaertr, IW.HG, Icairns, IceKarma, IncognitoErgoSum, Ioscius, Itai, Ivanov id, J.delanoy, J04n, JForget, JFreeman, JLaTondre, JNW, JaGa, Jackrm, Jafet, JakeVortex, JamesBWatson, Jauhienij, Jay Litman, Jdtyler, Jeames, Jeepday, Jeeves, Jeff Mortimer, Jeffq, Jennavecia, Jesse0986, Jfdwolff, Jgritz, Jgwales, Jhsounds, Jim Douglas, Jimp, JinJian, Jmh649, Joanneralph, John254, Jpbowen, Jpgordon, Julesd, Jumping cheese, Jusdafax, K.C. Tang, Kael, Katalaveno, Kbolino, Keegscee, Kevin Saff, Kikodawgzzz, Klichka, KnowledgeOfSelf, Koc91, Kslain, Kuru, KyraVixen, Kzhr, LOL, LadyofShalott, Ladyofwisdom, Lazerxplosion, Ledzeppelin463, Ligulem, LinDrug, Lipothymia, LowVision, Lucky55399, Lyght, Lyndsayruell, MJOLNIRchief90, MSTCrazy, Madeleine, Malcolm Farmer, Maniwar, Marek69, Maria Sieglinda von Nudeldorf, MarkSweep, Marnanel, Marokwitz, Martin-C, Master of Puppets, MaxSem, Maxis ftw, Mayooranathan, Meelar, Mentifisto, Mephistophelian, Metricopolus, Michael Hardy, Michaeldsuarez, Micki, Mijt, Mike1feguard, Mild Bill Hiccup, Mina mage, Mintgus tennis club, Minnaert, Mo0, Moink, MojoTas, Moshe Constantine Hassan Al-Silverburg, MrOllie, Ms2ger, Msljy, Mufka, Mwanner, Mysid, N2e, NawlinWiki, Neko-chan, Neochica88, Neverquick, Nifky?, Nlu, NoahB, NorthernThunder, Nu7i, NyAp, Obli, Oda Mari, Omassey, Omicronpersei8, One Salient Oversight, Optho Raptor, Oren0, OrgasGirl, Orlandoturner, Osm agha, Ottawa4ever, Oxymoron83, Patrick, Patxi lurra, Pax85, Pedant, Persian Poet Gal, Peter Ellis, Pewwer42, Pharaoh of the Wizards, Philip Trueman, Piclover87, Pill, Pingveno, Pit, PoliceZ, Pompski89, Pork fried cat, Portalian, Precession, PrincessofLlyr, Prolog, Prophaniti, Pseudo daoist, Psychonaut, Punkymonkey987, Purpleice, Quadell, Quintote, Quirkie, R'n'B, RDBrown, RFBailey, RJASE1, Raggedjoe, Rahm Kota, Ranveig, Ravizzle45, Rawling, Razimantv, Reach Out to the Truth, Recognizance, Rednuts devilpubes, Redsoxfreak000, RexNL, Reywas92, Rhobite, Rich Farmbrough, Rjwilmsi, Rmosler2100, Rnb, Rnorton215, Robinh, Roryshaughn, Rothorpe, Rtviper707, Ryan, Ryan Postlethwaite, S h i v a (Visnu), SM, Samsryed, Sanderbeil, Sarranduin, SatuSuro, Scarian, Scarps, Schekinov Alexey Victorovich, Scraggy4, Scymso, Sd31415, Sdoman, Sekiyu, Sepeople, Sfarrowsc, Shadowjams, Shanes, Shoeofdeath, SidP, Sillyfolkboy, Sir Sputnik, Sjakkalle, Slawojarek, Sligocki, Slowking Man, Smack, Smalljim, Smilesfoxwood, Smjg, Snideology, Spencerk, Spookfish, Staffwaterboy, Stefan da, Steinsky, Stephenb, Steve Murgaski, Stevenfruitsmaak, Su37amelia, Subdolous, Susan118, Swerdnaneb, T.roak67, Tarek, Tarquin, Tassedethe, Taylorlovesyou, Tejahb, The Anome, The Thing That Should Not Be, The Transhumanist, Thehelpfulone, Themfromspace, Thue, Tide rolls, Tim Starling, Tiptoety, Tirabo, ToNToNi, Tom Squire, Topbanana, Tregoweth, Trevor MacInnis, Troydlaplante, Tulpan, Twice25, Uncle Dick, Unknown W. Brackets, Unmitigated Success, Vaughan, Vegas Bleeds Neon, Vegaswikian, Venior, Versus22, Villy on Wheels, Vineeboy, Violetriga, Voyagerfan5761, Wavelength, Webber123, WhisperToMe, Will tad, Wimt, WojPob, Wtmitchell, Wuzzybaba, Xafifah, Xp54321, Xullius, YeaWyatt, Yidisheryid, Zafiroblue05, Zepheus, Zodon, Zzuuzz, ܡܝܟ, ಚಿ೯ಕಿ೮೫, 590 anonymous edits

Dystrophy *Source*: http://en.wikipedia.org/w/index.php?oldid=402946267 *Contributors*: AnjaManix, Bill, CopperKettle, DO11.10, Inferiority, Jasadbaefia, Jeff G., Kubanczyk, Kweeket, Leviel, Lisaharvey5, N2e, Nkayesmith, Radagast83, Skysmith, Viriditas, Why Not A Duck, 12 anonymous edits

Photoreceptor cell *Source*: http://en.wikipedia.org/w/index.php?oldid=412370708 *Contributors*: AED, Ambitiousboy, Appraiser, Arcadian, BD2412, Bensaccount, BobbyBoulders, Bomac, CDN99, Cam27, Canley, Citotoxico, ClockworkSoul, Closedmouth, Cybercobra, Delldot, Denis tarasov, Dicklyon, Download, Drybittermelon, Dual Freq, Excirial, Fangfufu, Enformatics, Giftlite, H2g2bob, Hodja Nasreddin, Hordaland, Icairns, Indolering, Jag123, Jjron, Just plain Bill, Kaihsu, KnightRider, Kosigrim, L Kensington, Lasseisan, Livick75, Lovemuffin333, Magioladitis, Magister Mathematicae, MartinSpacek, Materialscientist, Mikael Häggström, MollyNYC, NifCurator1, Nono64, Nrbelex, Nuno Tavares, Nuvitauy07, Nxtid, Ost316, Panek, Paskari, PhilKnight, Phtalo, Rbarreira, Rettetast, Rich257, Sakurambo, Sayeth, Sbierwagen, Science Study, Scott Coleman, Serpent's Choice, Slmader, Srleffler, Stemonitis, Stillnotelf, Tameeria, Tevildo, Theshadow27, Thue, Tupiac, Tjerman, TomViza, Tyłuma, Wickey-nl, Xhin, YUL89YYZ, Yuckfoo, 81 anonymous edits

Retinal pigment epithelium *Source*: http://en.wikipedia.org/w/index.php?oldid=412311417 *Contributors*: AED, Anassagora, Arcadian, Areosaf, C4 Diesel, Caerwine, ClementChesnin, CopperKettle, Groogle, Gustavocarra, Jfdwolff, Minimac, Nuvitauy07, Pekaje, Riana, Richerman, SF007, Una Smith, Walimania, 17 anonymous edits

Retina *Source*: http://en.wikipedia.org/w/index.php?oldid=412311417 *Contributors*: AED, Aboriginal Noise, AcademyAD, Acdx, Alasdair, Aleator, Alex, Alexei Kouprianov, Anaxial, Ancheta Wis, Andre Engels, Angela, Angevin1117, Aquilosion, Arcadian, AxelBoldt, Badjoby, Bcebul, Bentu, Bernard Teo, BoP, Bobblewik, Borofkin, Bosox5 2000, Burwellian, CALR, CLW, Caltrop, Carfinder, Cfaikle, Chadroemer, CliffC, Coelacan, CopperKettle, CosineKitty, Ceason, Cureden, Cybernautdoc, DanMS, David Berson, Delldot, Delta G, Deor, Diannaa, Diberri, DrBob, Duffman, Dysmorodrepanis, EJSawyer, Eestickler, Elassint, Emperorbma, Everyking, Felixboy, Fæ, Gadfium, Gaelle Desbordes, Ggem, Giftlite, Gilliam, Gogo Dodo, Gracefool, Gradenko, Hauskalainen, Hecko X, Heidimo, HendrixEesti, Heron, HitamHangus, Hordaland, Hunt9, Iago Dali, Inka 888, Irdepesca572, Iriss, J. Spencer, J.e, Jackl69007, Jaesim25, James Callahan, Jamesday, Jauerback, Jerzy, Jfdwolff, Jmundo, Jobe layton, Joelmills, John Cardinal, JohnJohn, John Lattier, Johnkarp, KFP, Kanags, Karenjc, Kate, Kkgrf1234, KnowledgeOfSelf, Knutux, Korath, Kpjas, Kubigula, Kubra, Leuqarte, LibLord, Liftarn, Lilmike121, Little Mountain 5, LittleHow, Local2remote10, Lpireyn, Luk, MCTales, MKR, Malo, Martinus, Martynas Patasius, Matusz, Meduz, Megaboz, Melaen, Mikael Häggström, Mlaffs, Morganfitzp, MrZap, Myanw, Myscrnnn, Naddy, NawlinWiki, Nono64, Nuvitauy07, Oli Filth, Olivier, Omegatron, Omicronpersei8, Paskari, Pinky sl, Prat, Prashanthns, Puffin, Radomir, Radon210, Raul654, Rich Farmbrough, Rjwilmsi, Robby miles, Robert P. O'Shea, Rolypolyman, RoyBoy, Rsabbatini, S0me 10ser, SF007, Sayeth, Sbharris, Sciurinæ, Seabhcan, Sfdyst, Sir Tanx, Slmader, SpeedBump, Stillnotelf, SuperHamster, Superblood7, Sushi, Susurrus, Svick, Szquirrel, Tabletop, Tatarize, Template namespace initialisation script, The Anome, The wub, The-tenth-zdog, The.Filsouf, TheCoffee, Thesoxlost, Thinng, TimBentley, TimVickers, Timekop, Tnxman307, TonyW, TwoOneTwo, UK Records, Utcursch, VMS Mosaic, Wa0rse, Wandell, Wavelength, Wesley1610, WikipedianProlific, Wilke, Wood Thrush, Wwwwwwwwwoooooowww, ...

Xoneca, Yamamoto Ichiro, Yekrats, Zzuuzz, आरोग्य भारताण, 270 anonymous edits

Peripheral vision *Source*: http://en.wikipedia.org/w/index.php?oldid=411680927 *Contributors*: 27 Juni, AED, Ahunt, Alphachimp, Antandrus, Antilived, Bonslywizard, Brilliant Pebble, Cleared as filed, DMahalko, Danski14, DeadRook, Debresser, Difu Wu, Discospinster, Duncan, Eagleal, Edward321, Fastilysock, Gamma1847, Gogo Dodo, GoingBatty, Graft, Hans-Werner34, Hunterfisher, IRP, Immunize, InvictaHOG, Jusdafax, Killiondude, Kingpomba, Kubigula, Kurtilein, Lbgrowl, LeaveSleaves, LilHelpa, Mattlencfc, Mr.Yahoo!, NawlinWiki, Oxymoron83, PBP, Ralphwiggam75, Recognizance, Res2216firestar, Richard001, Riotrocket8676, Rjwilmsi, Roland299, Ronhjones, Scarian, Shard Heilia, Signalhead, SimonP, Slysplace, SpencerWilson, Steve Bearman, Stuz, Sum0, The Thing That Should Not Be, Thrissel, Tide rolls, Tommymine1525, Tony1, Trelawnie, Twinsday, Wakablogger2, Whoelius, Woohookitty, 126 anonymous edits

Degenerative disease *Source*: http://en.wikipedia.org/w/index.php?oldid=400795765 *Contributors*: 16@r, Akerans, Alansohn, BTLizard, Contributor777, Craig Pemberton, Cyborg Ninja, Diannaa, Drgarden, Eldur Vindr, Fences and windows, Jfdwolff, Justc001, Jóna Þórunn, Leeearnest, Mhsb, Nihiltres, Not Particularly Smart, R500Mom, Sintaku, Sjsilverman, Taopman, The Literate Engineer, Tide rolls, Transhumanist, Varano, Wideg3cko, Yosri, 32 anonymous edits

Image Sources, Licenses and Contributors

License